DATE DUE

OC 21 '93			
JE 17 '94			
SE 30 '94			
JY 22 '98			
JA 9 '99			
MAR 2 9 2001			
JE 2 '05			

DEMCO 38-296

You and Your Clients: Human Relations for Cosmetology

You and Your Clients: Human Relations for Cosmetology

by Leslie Edgerton

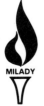

Milady Publishing Company
(A Division of Delmar Publishers Inc.)
Two Computer Drive West, Box 12519
Albany, New York 12212

Editor: Catherine Frangie

Photographer: Elizabeth Clester

Cover Photographer Steven Landis
Cover shot on Location at the Nardi Salon, NYC

Illustrator: Shiz Horii

Copyright © 1992
Milady Publishing Company
(A Division of Delmar Publishers Inc.)

Printed in the United States of America

10 9 8 7 6 5 4 3 2 1

ISBN

Library of Congress Cataloging-in-Publication Data

Edgerton, Leslie.
    You and your clients: human relations for cosmetology / by Leslie
Edgerton.
        p.   cm.
    ISBN 1-56253-058-5
    1. Beauty shops—Management. 2. Interpersonal relations.
    I. Title.
    TT965.E33   1992
    746.7'2'0688—dc20

                                                          90-27866
                                                               CIP

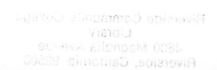

DEDICATION

Once in a lifetime, if you're very lucky, comes along a person who illuminates every corner of your world, puts a spring into your step, and makes you anxious to greet each new day, and who, just by being part of your universe, makes that experience a joyful and glad one. Such a person is my wife and partner, Mary Frances Edgerton, who is the source of my inspiration not only for this book, but also for most of my life. Without her, this humble effort would lie here undone, and the rest of my world would have a little duller color, a little less fire.

There are three other people who deserve my thanks: Britney, Sienna, and Mike, who allowed me to sacrifice our time together to complete this book. Thanks, kids. I love you.

ACKNOWLEDGMENTS

Although my name appears as author of this book, it could not have been written without the help of many people. Chief among them are my photographer ''Liz'' Clester; the models who gave us their time; and my wife and fellow hairstylist, Mary, who took care of our son Michael and my daughters Britney and Sienna during the long hours it took to actually write the book. Helpful suggestions came to me from Thia Masciana, Educational Director for the International Color Exchange, who played a large part in the sections on hair coloring and your client. Another source of valuable information was provided by Lois Shirley, the Artistic Director for the Regis Salon at Nieman-Marcus in Houston, Texas. And, of course, none of this would be possible without the divine guidance and inspiration provided by my editor, Catherine Frangie, and her able assistant editor Jacqueline Flynn, without whom I would still be trying to figure out how to do this!

TABLE OF CONTENTS

Introduction

Many years ago, during the height of the Vietnam War and shortly after being honorably discharged from the U.S. Navy, I picked up my first pair of scissors and cut my first head of hair. I can't remember who that first poor soul was, but I am reasonably certain his or her haircut didn't approach the quality of craftsmanship my most recent one has!

Some of you undoubtedly knew from early on that you wanted to be hairdressers, but I know many of you who are my peers in this wonderful business of creating beauty for others who would never have dreamed in a million years that this would be the way you would be earning a living. I certainly didn't! I didn't know exactly what it was I would be when I "grew up," but perming hair was not only not high on my list—it wasn't even *on* my list! I had this half-focused idea that I was destined to become the next Hemingway or J. D. Salinger. In the meantime I kept my body and soul together with a variety of jobs, none of which excited me enough to continue them for very long. I worked in an iron foundry, as a welder, in a grocery store, selling insurance, recruiting electronics engineers as a *headhunter;* my own personal list of *careers* goes on and on. Nothing satisfied me, until one day, a friend made a suggestion that would lead me to the niche in life that would not only satisfy the creative juices that bubbled and boiled within, but would also feed the hunger I had for social contact with other human beings.

He suggested I try cutting hair.

Notice I said "cutting hair"; not "becoming a hairdresser." Or a "hair designer." Or a "stylist." Not that there's anything wrong with any of those designations; the term I prefer currently is *hair designer,* but being known as a *hair cutter* is profoundly honorable and is what we do, primarily.

Once I had (nervously) attempted (and completed) my first haircut, I knew then that this was what I had always wanted to do. More than anything else I had ever been exposed to, this vocation of making others beautiful or handsome satisfied virtually all the requirements that, for me, my life's work would have to do to make me happy.

And so it has, since 1966, when I made my first tentative snip.

It has also enabled me to enjoy a very nice lifestyle, earning a very handsome income.

It has allowed me to meet and talk with people from all walks of life, from those whose names would be familiar to everyone in the country, to those whose names are only known to a small group of friends and family, but who are, nonetheless, every bit as fascinating as the more famous clients I have been privileged to serve.

It has allowed me to work all over the United States and earn a good income immediately upon moving to a new area or state. It has given me respect among those whom I meet, whether socially or professionally. It has kept my mind alert by learning the new techniques and styles that change almost daily. It has kept me young at heart and in my soul. It has given me back far more than I have taken from it. This is one great vocation, this cutting of the hair! Which brings us to the point of this book.

One of the observations I have made over the years, in various locales and salons, is a sad one. Sad, in that it need not be this way.

Wherever I have worked, in big towns, small towns, sophisticated salons, everyday shops, East Coast, West Coast, Midwest, or South, the tragic fact keeps reappearing and it is this: *Twenty percent of the salons do eighty percent of the business.* And, conversely, *eighty percent of the remaining salons fight over the remaining twenty percent of the business.* From the tiny village of Lakeville, Indiana, where I began my career, to the biggest and most sophisticated salons in New Orleans and southern California, the shakeout remains the same.

Why such a disparity? Why do a minority of hairdressers amass the lion's share of the hairstyling dollars?

It's not ability. It's not salon cleanliness. It's not more favorable locations. It's not relative politeness or rudeness to clients. It's not attractiveness of furnishings or the *look* of the salon. All of those things and many others are obviously important, but they are not the cause of the disparity.

One thing, and one thing only, separates the busy salon and stylist from the ones that are not: Communication—or, *mis*communication—between stylist and the client in the chair. That's it. It's that simple. It's the *Key to Success.*

I have seen hairstylists become very successful and enjoy a solid booking schedule, in the face of such obstacles as lack of outstanding talent and ability on their part; a dirty salon; poor location; inconvenient accessability; run-down equipment; a rude or incompetent receptionist; and a hundred and one other supposed *obstacles.* These factors are obstacles, certainly, but more often than not, are used as *alibis,* or reasons the hairdresser gives herself for not being busy.

Communication is the *Key to Success.*

And that's what this book will do for you: not only show you the importance of proper communication, but also give you concrete methods to better those skills. When you begin communicating effectively, your self-esteem will begin to rise, the respect you enjoy from your clients and others will begin to rise, and a curious thing will happen; your appointment book will begin to fill up, days and weeks ahead.

Each of us has a *TV* set in our heads. The client that sits in your chair also has such a TV set. The whole trick is to get both you and your client tuned in to the same channel with a clear, sharp picture.

And this is what we're about to learn. How to tune our TV sets. It will be fun learning and the payoff is enormous.

Let's begin!

CHAPTER 1

Ambiguous Terms:
How to Reach Common Definitions—The *Crux* of the Communication Problem

CHAPTER LEARNING OBJECTIVES

The stylist successfully mastering this chapter will know:

1. *The chief reason we miscommunicate.*
2. *The importance of proper communication.*
3. *Whom you need to communicate with.*
4. *How to "fix" our professional language.*
5. *Tuning our mental "TV sets."*
6. *Using video and television as communication aids.*

The primary factor at the core of nearly every salon failure, and the chief reason we as stylists fail to build a solid, profitable following, is simply that of poor communication. We are either not taught good communication skills or have not learned their importance in achieving success in our profession. We focus so much time, energy, and effort into developing technical skills and expertise and relegate the art of effective communication to a lesser role. In reality, however, aligning our thoughts with those of our clients is probably the single most important skill that can be learned.

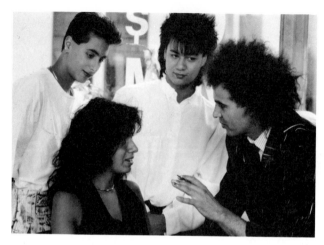

Fig. 1.1

The principal reason we can't talk to each other effectively, stylist-to-client, is that we don't have a proper language with which to do so, i.e., a common, mutually understandable language.

In any other endeavor, discipline, science, or study, there exists a special language for that field. All physicists, for example, agree upon a common definition for the word *neutron*. The word neutron conjures up the same exact mental picture for all those so engaged in the study of physics, regardless of the school at which they studied, or even their native languages, and it is thus that they are able to communicate. They possess a common language, and from this common language, are able to discuss intelligently their science with each other and to understand readily what the other is saying. This is the basis for all communication.

Oh, certainly, we have a *language*. We have special words in our lexicon also. Let me give you one: *short*. As in, "I'd like my hair cut *short*." Do you know what that means? I don't. I suspect many others don't either. Or, let's take another term used frequently in the styling business: *loose curl*. Do you know what a *loose curl* is? I'm under the impression I do—it's when you use a purple or larger perm rod. But, then, I have friends who swear a loose curl is achieved with using a gray or white perm rod. I'll wager that if I were to pick ten stylists from ten different salons, or even ten people from the street at random and ask them to tell me what they believe a loose curl looks like, I'd be fortunate to find three in either group that would pick the same-sized rod that I or you would.

It quickly becomes evident where most of our communication problems stem from. We simply don't have a common language with definite words and terms that are crystal clear to everyone. We have a *language,* such as it is. Most of us have a personal definition of the word *short,* and most of us can visualize a mental picture of a *loose curl,* but the difficulty lies in the generalness and vagueness of the words we use. And words without sharply defined and universally accepted meanings are nothing more than sounds we utter, and of little use in communicating, except poorly.

However, a neutron is a neutron. Period. It is not to be confused with an *ion* or a *neuron* or anything else but another neutron. The physicist sees but one thing in his or her mind. *Short,* on the other hand, has a thousand different meanings. Short, to the girl who can sit on her hair means something drastically different from what it means to the girl who has a short wedge. See? Take that last sentence, for example. How would you define a *short wedge?* Whew! Now, we've got *two* terms to define! Is a short wedge one that hits the collar? Is it one that is three inches above the collar? Is the weight line at the occipital bone? Or is it lower, at the bottom perimeter of the haircut?

Early on in my own career, cutting and styling hair at Michael and Company, in South Bend, Indiana, I had developed into something of a *hotshot,* a curious disease that strikes many young, too-soon-successful hairstylists. I had enjoyed heady success in styling competitions, having just won a second and third place in the Indiana State Styling Championships, on my first attempt, in the Lady's Fashion Cut and the Men's Cut Divisions. I enjoyed a full booking in the salon and labored under the delusion that Vidal Sassoon could pick up a few tips from watching me work. Michael and Company just happened to be the most progressive salon in town as well as one of the more forward-thinking salons in the entire Midwest. They still enjoy that distinction today, over two decades hence.

My swollen ego hid from me the fact that any personal success was derived from where I was. I had come on board with a zero client base and was so ignorant that I did not even know how to do a simple cut such as a *shag,* which happened to be the hot style of the moment and the one we performed on the great majority of our clients. The full booking I enjoyed immediately was not related to any great talent of my own; rather, it was merely the overflow from the other stylists in the salon who were tremendously busy.

I remember as if it were yesterday, laboring for over two hours on my first *style*—a shag layer cut. I would stop every few minutes to watch the stylists on either side of me who were cutting the same style (much faster!) and attempt to imitate what they were doing. Somehow, I got the cut completed, and it must not have been too horrible because the client paid.

The point is, I came aboard with nothing and received not only a full booking right away, but also some of the best training available anywhere at the time. It was because of the intense training I received that I was able to do so well in my first styling competition.

It was during this period that a new client seated herself in my chair and asked for a *body wave*. Being the progressive stylist I fancied myself to be, I proceeded to give her a beautiful permanent wave, using purple rods. After rinsing the neutralizer and combing through her hair, I proudly displayed her gorgeous loose curl to her, upon which she wailed, "There's no curl!" Well, there *was*, at least in my mind and according to our salon's definition of *body* or *loose* curl. The only problem was, *our* definition didn't fit *her* definition.

All her life she had received perms given on blue, yellow, or small pink rods, and the size of the curl the large purple rods gave her appeared almost nonexistent to her eye. That was 1968, and she had only recently given up wetsetting her hair and turned to blow-dried styles. The curls a gray or white rod would have given her would have been loose to her, which to me would have seemed tight.

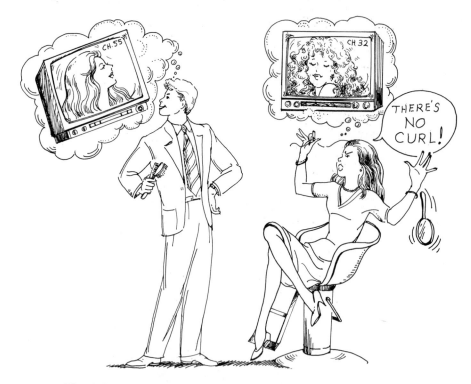

Fig. 1.2 Two different television channels.

I was devastated. And mad. Didn't she realize she had just been given the best perm possible from the best permer possible?

I'm sure I kicked something in the back room. I then took my sad tale of woe to Michael Murray, the owner and chief stylist, and, who remains today, one of the most innovative and creative stylists I have ever been privileged to work for. I fully expected him to commiserate with me, but he did something wholly unexpected.

He went back out to my client and apologized to her! Not only that, he told her she could either not pay at all, or return and either have me give her another perm with tighter curl or have another stylist do so.

I was crushed! I felt like quitting and going back to something less demanding, like brain surgery. My boss, my hero, had taken a client's side against mine when I was in the right! Purple rods fit the salon's definition of loose curl. Why had he done this?

And then, I did the only intelligent thing I had done that day. I listened to Michael. He explained that, yes, the curl you obtained from a purple rod was a *loose* curl, and was what we defined loose curl to be. However, he said, it obviously didn't fit my *client's* definition, and *it was my client's definition that counted,* not the salon's definition, or mine. This was a new concept for me and the beginning of my real education. This knowledge was to prove more useful to me in building my career than learning twenty new cuts!

It was my first lesson in communication. Thank goodness it sank in!

My TV set wasn't tuned to the same channel as my client's. I was on channel 55 when she was on channel 32.

What I had done, under the attitude I held, was what many of us in hairstyling do each and every day. I simply failed to communicate.

As we have seen, the terms we use and the words we employ are at the crux of the communication problem.

How then, do we get around this problem? By inventing new words and assigning them exact definitions? That *might* work, but do you honestly believe you could get six hundred thousand hairdressers as well as millions of clients to agree to a whole new vocabulary? And roughly six minutes after the new words would be brought out, the definitions would begin to change, and then new words would be introduced, along with the latest style, and then . . .

So, it seems that particular solution appears more than a bit impractical and unworkable. Is there any answer then?

Sure there is!

We can use the words we already have, the *shorts,* the *loose curls,* the *layer the tops,* and tighten up the definitions with various aids. Remember, it's not important that *everyone* in the galaxy understand and agree with our terms and

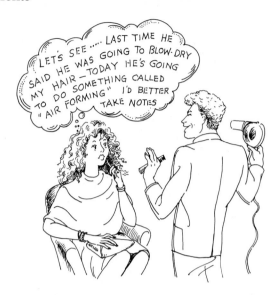

Fig. 1.3 A brave new world and vocabulary.

definitions—it's only important that *two* people do—*you and your client*. The more we can tighten the definition and clarify the concept we happen to be discussing with our client, the closer we come to sharing the same mental picture on our internal TV screens. All we ever have to worry about educating are those two people: you and the client seated before you.

Before you make the first tiny snip, or put the first perm rod in the hair; before you even begin to think about mixing up that bowl of color in the back room—be absolutely certain that both TV sets, yours and your client's, are tuned to the same channel and that the picture is as clear as you can possibly make it. Remember also that *you* are the tuner, not the client. It is *your* responsibility to take charge of the communication, not the clients'. The more you perfect your ability to communicate with your clients, the higher your success level will climb; and that success can be visibly measured not only in increased client satisfaction, but also in the number of clients you begin to see and in the size of the check you receive at the end of the week.

The highest paid hairdressers are sometimes not even those who have the most talent or the highest technical ability. Isn't that surprising? Sometimes they are, but many times they're not. But one thing they are the best at is that all successful hairstylists share the ability to communicate with the client so that (1) both *see* the finished result before the work is begun, and (2) the finished result matches the expectations.

Here's another example of miscommunication, on a more everyday level. When a friend tells you she took a *cab* to work this morning, you have a mental picture of the vehicle she traveled in. You are thus communicating. You are talking to each other and understanding clearly what the other means. If, on the other hand, your friend told you that she came to work in a *hoxie,* you would stare at her as if she had just swallowed rat poison, and you might even make a crack about her mental state. Or, assuming you are of a more polite nature, you might inquire as to just exactly what a *hoxie* is. If you didn't ask, and you hadn't a clue as to what a *hoxie* is then you weren't communicating. Only one of you has the definition, and to communicate effectively, both of you must have the same definition, or at least be fairly close to the same understanding of what the word or term used means.

This is, sadly, what occurs in hair salons every day of the week. It is the single most common reason that we, as stylists, don't deliver to the client what the client has in mind, and it is the single most common reason we don't see that client the second time.

We are *failing to bridge the gap between the style the client wants and the style the client gets.*

Remember this: *Clients are on a safari to discover the stylist who sees the same mental image that they themselves see.* Don't you want to be at the end of that safari?

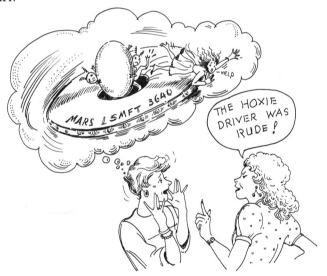

Fig. 1.4 Define the terms you use when communicating; otherwise, you can't be understood.

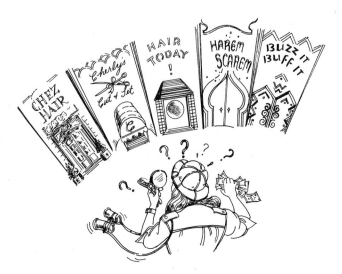

Fig. 1.5 The great client safari.

Another obstacle to effective communication is our ego. Many times, we are working overtime to convince the client that *our* vision of what the client should wear is the only proper one, and we sometimes don't take into account or pay attention to what the client's own wants are. Learn to listen to what your client is telling you. Many of the people who have sat down in my chair have told me that "You are the first person who did what *I* wanted." When you hear clients say things like that, over and over, you begin to get a clue as to why many stylists sit staring into their mirrors large portions of their work week.

There is a fine line between being a waiter or waitress and merely taking the client's *order* . . . and being a true *professional,* highly trained and up-to-date, knowing exactly what looks best on the client and telling the client so. Yes, you *are* the professional, and yes, you do have a higher sense of what the client will look best in, but when push comes to shove, the only opinion that should win is the client's.

When you become argumentative with the lady or gentleman seated before you, insisting that their ideas are hogwash and only *you* know what is best for them, you have become counterproductive and have probably alienated the client to the point where he or she won't be back. Work to develop a sense of knowing when to back off in a disagreement and comply (cheerfully!) with the client, and your client return ratio will increase immensely.

There have been many times when I have found myself at odds with the client's wishes, and when those occasions arose, I would try not to be offensive in giving the client my rationale as to why she should follow my suggestions, but, in the final analysis, she got what *she* wanted and the service was not performed grudgingly, but with a positive frame of mind. Always keep in mind that it's the *client's* hair and it's the *client's* money—*she's* the one who has to wear the look you give her and she's the one that has to pay you for it.

There is the other side of the coin in instances such as these as well. When a client insists on a style that you know to be utterly wrong for her, or if she insists upon something so hideous and horrible you can't bear to have your *name* on it, or if she insists on a technique you know to be damaging to her hair physically, then you certainly have the right to refuse to perform the service. This should be done diplomatically so that both parties' dignity are preserved intact, but at times it may become necessary.

Only once have I refused to perform a style on a client. The style she insisted on so adamantly was the most outdated, outlandish look imaginable. I tried to convince her that what she wanted was not a wise choice, but she continued to insist that was what she wanted. I ended up telling her very politely that I couldn't, in good conscience, let her leave with the look she wanted, but that I knew a stylist who *did* perform the type of style she sought and did a good job and I would be more than happy to call the stylist myself and make an appointment for her. I didn't denigrate her decision or her choice whatsoever. I did explain to her that it violated my own sense of style, but that one's sense of style was a subjective one and only valuable to the person holding that view and the others sharing it, and that her own sense was not worse than mine, only different; that both had value.

She was pleased at the way I handled the "confrontation," and allowed me to make the appointment for her. I made certain she knew I respected her opinion even though I didn't share it, and we parted amicably. As she left, I made the suggestion that if she should change her mind in the future and decide to switch to the look I had suggested, that she allow me to do it for her. To my delight and surprise, about three months later, she phoned and made an appointment and allowed me to cut the style I had wanted.

The point is, I respected her and conducted the conversation in such a way that she respected me as well, and there were no ruffled feelings or wounded pride on either side. She wasn't made to feel stupid and consequently she became a client.

I am going to repeat this because it's so important: *Clients are on a safari to discover the stylist who sees the same mental image that they see.*

Now, I know you know what communication is, and you perhaps don't need an object lesson to learn about something you've been doing all your life, but, we both know that many times all of us forget the basic rules of communication: *Define the words and terms we commonly employ between each other.*

The first such means to sharpen the shared mental images you are trying to share is obviously visual. Chapter 5 delves into various effective ways to use pictures and other optical and visual aids. You will find it extremely useful.

There are other methods to achieve clarity in the language. One to be aware of at all times and to begin to employ now, is to clarify common terms already used. If possible, try to get the other stylists in your salon on the same page as well. The wider the circle of effective communicators becomes, the easier and better everyone begins to become clear to each other.

For example, I do a lot of color work in my salon. I worked as a platform artist for a major international color company for several years and the experience *turned me on* to the excitement to be obtained using color in its hundreds of ways.

Many times, I have had a client come to me and ask to have her hair *highlighted.* Usually, she was talking about lightening a small percentage of her hair by various means, foil or cellophane weaves and slices, or cap highlights. This is an area in which communication is doubly important. Sometimes what the client visualized in her mind was not what I would have considered a highlight, but more properly a *blonding,* or almost a complete color change. My personal definition of a highlight is that it is a process by various means and methods whereby you *subtly* brighten existing hair color and make it come alive. My definition of a successful highlight is when a friend of the client says, "Oh, your hair looks great!" and doesn't notice that it's been highlighted, only that it looks better than the last time she saw her. When another person says to that client, "Oh, your hair's been highlighted, hasn't it?" that's an unsuccessful highlight.

Now, that doesn't mean that my definition is the only right one; it's only *my* definition. *Mine and my client's.*

If I service a client who asks for a highlight and through discussion and observance, I determine what she really wants is not a highlight according to my definition, but what I would term a *blonding,* I take the time to explain the difference. Not that one is better than the other; there is no such value, but to simply begin to establish accurately the terms we will use with each other. If she, indeed, desires a blonding, then I will certainly and cheerfully give her what she desires, but I want both of us to use the same term for it.

It may seem easier to just ignore whatever term she is using and give her what she wants without comment, but the more you do that, the more you muddy up the language and the less effective in communicating you become.

Many of the terms we use are as sloppy as the above example, and because we haven't taken the time to clarify our terms, they become less and less clear to more and more people, thereby losing any effectiveness or value in communicating. Being dilligent about getting together on the terminology between you and your clients will eventually result in easier and clearer communication, thereby saving time (which is money, the rumor goes!), and getting closer and closer to giving all of our clients what they desire.

It is up to you to create the language used.

In the case of permanent waves and resultant curl size, a tremendous source of miscommunication, I have found a great aid to be my Perm Book. My Perm Book is simply a photo album filled with Polaroid shots of clients after a fresh perm, photos taken after the final rinse, while the hair is combed out and wet, *before it is styled and dried.* It shows simply, combed-out, wet, freshly permed hair, usually taken from the rear to show a good sample of the hair. I have long hair, short hair, blonde hair, red hair, fine hair, thick hair, every kind of hair except mohair for each rod size. I have done the same with a book of highlighted hair, except that the highlighted hair photos (which include all degrees of highlighting as well as samples of carmelizings, color scrunchings, shoeshining, dimensional color effects, and other techniques) are of styled and finished hairstyles. An invaluable communication aid!

With my Perm Book, I can go to a client and say, "This is what size curl your hair will obtain if I use a peach-colored rod." Or an orange rod. Or whatever.

With my color book (which I title "Les and Mary's Coloring Book," Mary being my partner in life and business), I can show a client what I consider a true *highlight* and point out the difference between that and a heavier effect, or a *blonding,* thereby saving a serious instance of miscommunication. Inexpensive to create, such photo albums are invaluable aids and very powerful tools in establishing clear and concise communication.

In my Perm Book, I attempt to show as many lengths, styles, colors, and textures of hair as possible with each rod size, so the client can see that the curl from a brown rod will look differently on six-inch-long black hair than it will on thirty-six-inch-long strawberry blonde hair. Many of the perm photos have a wet shot and then the finished look next to it.

These are just a couple of examples of ways in which you can create, at very little cost, your own very effective visual aids.

Videotapes offer other intriguing possibilities. Many tapes are available from product manufacturers and show scores of current styles, and if you have your own video camera, you can create your own personal catalog of perm effects, color effects, or hairstyles. The new generation of video programs allow you to do the same.

Speaking of video, this is a relatively new area that has been largely untapped by many in our profession. The surface has just begun to be scratched, and the outlook is rosy for the future of video. Eventually, video will play a significant part in every aspect of the salon business, just as computers have.

For example, in our own salon, "Bold Strokes Hair Designers," we use video in a number of ways, and almost daily it seems, someone in the salon comes up with a new and inventive way to expand our uses.

We have a videotape we prepared ourselves that is a fifteen-minute film in which we explain to a new client what our philosophy is and what services we offer. We are preparing a tape for our hair-replacement department that will show our male clientele the possibilities of hairpieces.

We carry a large number of retail product lines, and in several of our main lines, we have a small black and white TV that is situated at the end of the aisle that continually plays a product information tape the manufacturer provides to us. Some manufacturers also provide a *computer* that allows customers to ask it questions about their hair and then prescribes a regimen of cleansing and styling aids that will best suit the client's needs. We have such a unit that supplies data on three major product lines, and it has made those lines the top sellers of all our twenty-plus brands.

We have a large television set in the reception area on which are continually played haircutting and styling tapes. This stimulates a great deal of interest in new hairstyles, thereby not only creating new and additional business, but also enhancing our image as being on the cutting edge of fashion and technology.

We are in the process of putting video cameras in the salon, trained on the styling stations, where we will film various clients (with their permission) who have a style we think attractive, and the video will show on a wide-screen TV in our street-side window to passersby.

We have also created other tapes to be used in consultations. Along with our men's hair replacement tape, we show tapes on braiding, hair extensions, color and perm techniques, and one on home hair care, giving easy styling tips. Each Tuesday evening, our newer stylists host a free blow-drying clinic for the public, which is a tremendous source of new clients for them, and at the beginning of the presentation, the home hair care tape is shown. The free blow-drying clinic is probably our biggest single source of new clients and details of how it is done are outlined in detail in Chapter 11, "How to Build a Full Booking in Three Months or Less."

The education that is available on videotapes is staggering! It is easily the most significant change ever in our education with video's ability to bring anyone up-to-date literally overnight with what's happening in the world's fashion capitals. Today, you can be in the smallest town in the country and be doing styles that were just yesterday introduced in Rome or London!

Take the videotape recorder (VCR) out of the backroom and put it out in front where the clients can see it. Don't be too worried that they will see your tapes on cutting hair and be tempted to open up a salon next door to you and become your competitor. That has hardly ever happened, to my knowledge!

It will do two things. It will stimulate a high level of interest among your clients in their own hair and its possibilities, and it will establish in their minds that you are education-minded and on top of your craft.

These are just a few examples of the possibilities video can play in communication, and doubtless, as time marches forward, creative minds will discover even more ways to utilize the medium. Videotape and computerization are the wave of the future, and will soon be a necessary and integral part of every successful salon.

Although video, snapshots, photos, and other visual aids are effective in salon communication, verbal skills should be used as well. Sometimes, the look you wish to explain cannot be found in an existing picture. Perhaps you are creating a style that has never been attempted before, at least not in the way you visualize. "Trust me," is not something very many clients are anxious to hear; they've been the victims of "trust me" before, perhaps!

Even though a visual aid cannot be found for the new look you are proposing, and you are forced to rely mostly on language to paint a picture, try to avoid the more ambiguous of terms. To the lady with shoulder-length tresses you wish to shorten to the nape of her neck, give her a hand mirror and turn her around so she can see where the hair will fall. *Chin-length* hair means so much more to the client when she actually sees her hair at that length, than when she merely hears you describe it.

If you have any talent at drawing, you may sometimes need to sketch your idea. Even done crudely, such a drawing can be very helpful. If there are no pictures available of the style you have in mind, see if there are perhaps portions of the style that you can show to the client. Something similar to the sides may be in one magazine, the back may be in another, the top on yet another page. Time is valuable, and so you don't want to spend an hour assembling every square inch of a style via various photos, but two or three pictures can give at least a general overview.

Ask the client from time to time if she understands the information you are imparting to her. Let her know you *want* her to ask questions about anything that is unclear. Sometimes miscommunication results when only a small part of what you are explaining is misunderstood, and could have been cleared up with a simple question at the right time. Encourage the client's participation in the consultation.

We teach all of our clients how to achieve their style at home, quickly and easily (we utilize the KISS method—keep it simple, silly), and we have evolved an air-forming (our term for blow-drying) technique that works for almost every style. We have a video the client can rent at a nominal charge that shows her how to care for her hair, both in styling and for its health, and we encourage her to tape her own copy of it. During the styling session, we go so far as to even place the blow dryer and brush in the clients' hands, so we know they understand.

But even with all the detail and attention we spend with the client on this portion of their style, we know that they may not have fully mastered the technique. Before we release them from the chair, we tell them, "It is a fact that the average person forgets fifty percent of what she has learned within twenty-four hours. This doesn't mean you are dumb—it merely means you are human and in the same boat as the rest of us. If you wake up tomorrow and attempt to do what we have shown you and you don't get the results you should, just pick up the phone and call us. We'll *walk* you through the procedure on the phone, and chances are very good that you simply forgot a small part of what we did. Because everything builds on the last part, that is what is probably causing you to get a result different from last night's. That's usually all it takes to get you back on track. If not, then we'll make an appointment for you, shampoo your hair, and let *you* dry it, with our direction."

We tell this to each and every client, and it pays off handsomely. And yes, I've gotten calls from clients who woke up the next day and forgot how to do their hair. But it usually only takes a minute to run through the regimen, and they're back on track. And yes, I've had to bring clients back in and shampoo their hair and watch them dry it, correcting their mistakes, but not too often, and believe me, those clients go out of their way to tell their friends how we stand behind them! We actually and honestly feel our clients know more about hair in general than many professionals, because we educate them about every single facet of their hair.

There are hard and fast rules involved in every single aspect of hair, from cutting to air-forming, from perming to coloring, and the more rules one knows and understands, the more that person gets the same, consistent result, time after time. Many times we don't yet know the law or rule and that's why we get into trouble. No one knows all the laws, physical and otherwise, that deal with hair, and that is why our own education should never cease. When you're green you're growing . . . and when you're ripe you're rotten!

When you have a client that has problems with her hair, especially in air-forming it, keep this simple saying in mind. Simplify, simplify, simplify! Break down what she is doing into its elements, and then discover what she is doing wrong.

A valuable tip I learned in teaching clients care of their hairstyle, especially in air-forming, is to teach them to break down the system we teach the first time they attempt it.

"The first time you try this technique," I explain, "don't pick up the brush in one hand and the dryer in the other and face your mirror. Turn your dryer on and lay it down. Pick up the brush and put it into position. Then, pick up the dryer and use it. If you try a new motor skill such as this the first time, with brush in one hand and dryer in the other, you are going to get very frustrated. First of all, this is alien to you. Second, you are looking into a mirror and everything is backward. So, you have to look into this mirror and figure out what to do with each hand at the same time. If you break it down the first time and take a little bit more time, the coordination will come to you about the third or fourth step in the procedure and you will quickly become adept at the method."

Learn to see hair through the client's eyes instead of the eyes of a seasoned professional such as yourself. They don't have the training you do, nor the vantage point you have, standing in front of them.

Remember that also when you are explaining things to your clients. Terms you take for granted, they may be unfamiliar with, or have an entirely different definition of. If you use the word tapered to a client who has gone to a barber-stylist, she will have a different image of the result than the one you will have if you are a cosmetologist. Many of the terms used in the industry have different meanings to its practitioners.

Use every means available that can increase communication between you and your client. Tweak and tune both your TV sets until you are both on the same channel and seeing the same movie. If you do so, there will most definitely be a happy ending! In later chapters we will get into detail various methods that will help increase your ability to communicate. Work hard at sharpening definitions, use pictures, use videos, use crude drawings if you have to, but always remember—*do whatever it takes to get your client's TV set on the same channel as yours!* And get both sets tuned in *before you begin the service.*

REVIEW

1. *The chief reason we miscommunicate:* We don't have terms with fixed definitions, commonly accepted, understood, and agreed upon by everyone.
2. *The importance of proper communication:* Improper communication is the prime reason we end up with dissatisfied clients. We don't lose clients

because of dirty salons, rudeness, or even poor work, but because we haven't communicated properly. Cleanliness, politeness, and professional ability *are* important as well, but communication is *paramount.*

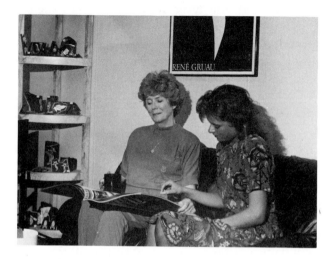

Fig. 1.6 Communication is the key to success.

3. *Who you need to communicate with:* Only one person; whoever is seated before you at the time.
4. *How to* fix *our professional language:* Use the terms we already employ, but clarify the definition. Use pictures, examples of persons you both know, prepared materials such as the *Perm Book;* in short, utilize anything and everything that can clarify the styling concept you are about to attempt.
5. *Tuning our mental TV sets:* Make certain your own TV set is tuned to the exact same channel as your client's. Don't be on channel 33 when she is watching the picture on channel 21!

CHAPTER 2

The Client *Talks* in Many Ways:

Sometimes What Someone "Says" Is *Not* What She Is "Saying"

CHAPTER LEARNING OBJECTIVES

The stylist successfully mastering this chapter will know:

1. *Individuals, many times, aren't communicating well with themselves.*
2. *How to recognize when what a person says verbally is not what they are really saying.*
3. *How to encourage such a client to show you what they really want.*

Assuming that what your client is saying to you is a true reflection of what she *sees* in her mind, is many times a false assumption. And you know what they say about the word *assume.*

We have all had the experience of the client who says she wants the "back shortened up to here" and indicates the length she wants by placing her hand on the back of her neck. And then we cut it to the length she pointed out and when the mirror was handed to her for her approval, and she went into cardiac arrest because you'd cut it six inches shorter than what she wanted. Even though she had shown you the length!

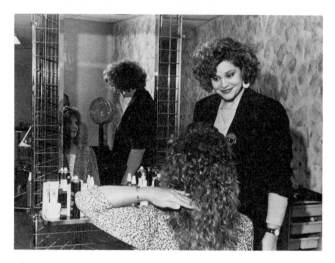

Fig. 2.1 "I just want a few inches off. About here, I think."

Or, the person who said she didn't want a "bob" even if you paid her a million dollars to do so, and then she described what she did want, and to you, her description sounded curiously close to what you and fifteen million others would call a "bob."

A great many people find it difficult, if not downright impossible, to describe properly what they want. And you thought hairstyling was going to be easy!

Years ago, in a misguided move, I briefly left the hairstyling profession for a stab at being a corporate raider, that profession that some call being a "recruiter" and others maybe more correctly term being a shark. After a while, I came to my senses and went back to doing what I did best, cutting, perming, and coloring hair, but during my temporary period of insanity, I was able to pick up some valuable lessons in human psychology. *People don't always say what they mean, even though they are convinced they do.*

For instance, while recruiting electronics engineers (EEs), one of the questions we asked was, "What do you view as your next career move or promotion?" Inevitably, the answer was, "Management." On the surface, that sounded all well and good, and the proper response—after all, *their* immediate superior was a manager, and naturally they felt that was the position they should be interested in. The first time I encountered this, I was excited, because I had just such a position to fill, and the engineer I was talking with was not only qualified (on paper) for the management position, but also seemed to feel it was what he wanted.

I burst into the office of my superior, Dick Pulse, of Kendall and Davis, Inc., to show him the excellent match I had made, mentally calculating how much of the agency fee I would be able to stick into my pocket once the deal was closed, and he asked to see the applicant's file.

He looked it over for all of ten seconds, handed it back, and said, "Don't send him to the interview. He doesn't want to be a manager."

Huh? Why on earth not, was the question that went through my mind, and Dick answered it.

"Look here at his job description. What does he do all day?"

That was easy. "He works with computers, designs things."

"Right. And what does he list for his interests and hobbies?"

"He has a home computer. He's a computer hack, likes to communicate with other computer hacks."

I still didn't get it, so Dick explained it in simple terms I could grasp.

"This guy's a *techy*. He enjoys things, not people. He works all day on a computer in a little room by himself and then goes home and plays with another computer. He's a *thing* person, not a *people* person. He'd be miserable in management."

We talked some more, and I began to see what he was saying. The applicant had done something we all do—he had miscommunicated with *himself!* In his mind, he was convinced he belonged behind a desk managing people, and this was what he had convinced himself he ought to be doing, but in reality he much more enjoyed working with his *machines*.

We were able to place him in a company that was employing a new concept (for the time) of providing parallel career paths for technical people. At the point where traditional tracking moved such a person into management, thereby many times attempting to place a square peg into a round hole, this corporation provided a technical track that was equal to the management track, but allowed the engineer to remain in research and design in a hands-on capacity.

What do engineers and recruiting have to do with hairstyling? Not much, ordinarily, except to illustrate an example of how many of our clients can be very intelligent otherwise, and fail to have a good understanding of what it is they really want.

Many times, that client who insists she wants a look the current hot rock star or movie actress is sporting, doesn't necessarily want that look at all, and will be unhappy once she receives it.

Your job is to discover what it is she's really after, and this isn't as difficult as it may seem. Sometimes the reason the client wants to look like some famous beauty is that a boyfriend or husband has suggested a resemblance, and human nature being what it is, the flattery works, giving her the desire to look even more like a recognized beauty. Reams of scientific psychological data have been accumulated that support such phenomenon, but that is far beyond our scope here. Suffice to say, such situations exist and although we don't have to have a thorough knowledge of the psychological reasons inherent, it is valuable to recognize such an instance when it occurs.

Whatever the appearance, all the client really wants is what most of us desire—to look more attractive. If you can show her how to accomplish this, you will have done your job and can accurately be called a *stylist*.

Don't try to probe too far into the depths of the client's psyche and figure out exactly what she is saying. It is sufficient only to know that she wants to look better than she has and proceed from there. Recognize that while her underlying reason for showing you a picture is to emerge from your salon looking better, consciously she has identified with the picture she is showing you, and diplomatically use that point to lead into what you would like to do for her.

For instance, you notice that the person in the picture has a square jaw similar to that of the client. Look for such similarities, for that is probably what she has keyed in on, also. You might begin the conversation by saying something like, ''That is a good choice to start from, Nancy. Both you and ___ have about the same jawline. See how she has more volume on the sides and how

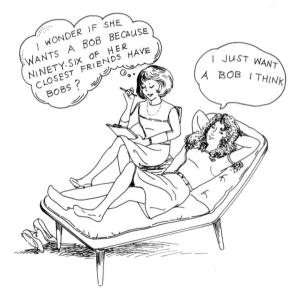

Fig. 2.2

the effect is to slim down the jaw? That's what I think you should also do, for the same reason. Now your texture and growth pattern are different, so it would be better to modify your look a bit—I think a body wave would be better to help you achieve the look you want. It will give you the same effect as ___ is able to achieve naturally. And the best thing is that although you'll be able to wear your hair in much the same way as ___ does, you'll also be able to achieve four or five other looks as well.''

A good idea to clue clients to when they bring in pictures, is to have them place their hand over the model's face and look just at the hairstyle, meanwhile picturing the same hair on their own head. Many times, the client doesn't realize she's looking at a sophisticated accumulation of many techniques, including professional camera lighting and equipment and painstaking makeup applications—not to mention that the artist assuredly selected the best model possible for the shoot. Many times when I have done a model's hair for hair and fashion magazines, I have used methods and techniques such as subtle backlighting or even wire harnesses to support and fill out the hairstyle, and as soon as the shoot was over, the hair collapsed. Chicanery perhaps, but if you think about it carefully, you'll realize that no one runs out into the street, grabs the first person that walks by, and takes their picture for a magazine.

You might bring this to the attention of your client and point out that sometimes the looks she sees in magazines are painstakingly crafted and many times aren't suited for practical, day-to-day wear.

Sometimes you may get a client who won't be talked out of looking exactly like the picture she is clutching, even though you know that there's no way in the world her hair would do that, and even if it did, she wouldn't look like the picture. Here is where all your tact and diplomacy will come into play. Quiz her about what it is she likes most about the picture or style. Usually, this is all that's needed to give you the necessary clue to what she's really seeing and relating to.

Above all, be truthful and honest with the client, although never to the point of insulting her. If she insists on looking like her friend Gail, whose hair you also do, point out that while yes, Gail looks terrific with the hair coming off her forehead and swept back, her own hair grows at a different angle and has a wholly different texture and therefore can't do what Gail's does, even with the same cut. Perhaps another service might help her achieve the look she's after, a permanent wave perhaps. Explain that if ten people have exactly the same cut, down to the *nth* centimeter, no two will look the same because of a myriad of factors, such as growth patterns, hair densities, hair colors, facial features and shapes, complexions, hair textures, and so on. Give her a way out by suggesting what you think she should let you do and give your reasons for your ideas.

Paint as accurate a portrait of the finished look as you can, along with the maintenance regimen required.

I recently had to discharge an employee who had only been with us for several weeks because he consistently refused to listen to what the client was really saying to him. My wife Mary and I both came to the same conclusion, that he suffered from some insecurities in his ability, and, therefore, compensated by attempting to always impose his will on his clients. We had several meetings with him and attempted to help him understand why clients were dissatisfied with his services and didn't return or demanded refunds. Neither Mary nor I enjoy discharging an employee, and we bend over backward to salvage such a situation, but this one particular stylist absolutely wouldn't listen to any of our suggestions and gave us no choice.

The last straw, the one that broke the proverbial camel's back, was when a client he had done the day previous, called back and asked to talk to the owner of the salon. Through her tears and gulps, I was able to ascertain that she had informed this particular stylist that she was to be married in four and a half months and wanted to let her shoulder-length hair grow out more to one length for the wedding ceremony. He proceeded to argue and cajole her into letting him layer the top drastically, insisting she was going to "love it"; it was the "latest thing," a new style he had just learned in a seminar. I happened to be in the vicinity at times while he styled her hair, and knew for a reasonable certainty that what she was telling me was pretty much the truth.

I had her come into the salon afterhours and examined her haircut. It was about as she had described, "hacked and chopped up." He had gone through every cutting instrument he possessed and some he borrowed to achieve this *masterpiece.* During almost every step of his cutting process he had also kept assuring her she was going to "love it," and that she should just "trust him," arguing volubly with her all along the way.

She had entered the salon in an imperial fashion—you know the type—and her attitude had intimidated him, so much that he grossly overcompensated by *proving* he was a great stylist by using every technique on her hair he had ever learned and by inventing some new methods heretofore unknown to any existing stylist. The result was an unmitigated disaster, the likes of which I had seldom been privy to.

I spent an hour with the young lady, showing her some styling methods she could use to *hide* the damage and reassuring her that her hair would grow out at least another four inches or more before the wedding. When she left, she was not only mollified and happy, but had become a loyal and trusting client of my own. She also left with a sizable check, the refund for her disastrous hair-

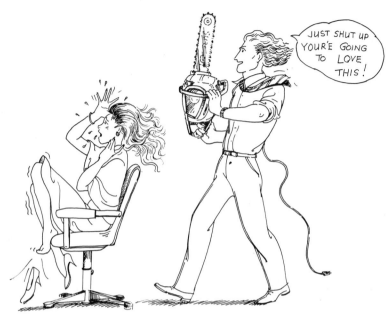

Fig. 2.3   Listen to the client and respect her wishes.

cut and the highlights he had also performed. There was nothing wrong with the highlights, but she got a full return anyway.

The next day, the stylist and I parted company. It was not because I had been forced to refund a client's money. That was not the first time that had happened, nor did I expect it to be the last. All of us, from time to time, create an unhappy client, even the best of us, and I have no quarrel with any stylist in my employ who gets into such a situation, provided he or she has performed properly and to the best of their ability. If there were such a thing as a perfect stylist, there would only be one salon and only one person working, and such is not the case. We all make mistakes, honest mistakes, but this was not an honest mistake by any means. He had been warned time after time, about just such instances, and had failed to comply, being thoroughly convinced his own sense of style was superior to the client's.

Such a stylist doesn't belong in our salon, and I trust, not in yours either.

This was a case in which the client had made a strightforward, simple request, and he had disregarded it. He couldn't even use the excuse that he had *misread* her; her request had been totally clear.

Listen to the client. Sometimes they are saying what they mean and sometimes they are not. Learn to distinguish between the two.

About a year ago, I got into trouble by not following my own advice. A new client, sent to me by another, informed me during the consultation, that she "didn't want a bob." She always received *bobs,* she said, from every stylist she ever went to, and she thought it made her look like an old lady. I wasn't too sharp that day, for if I had been, I would have realized that the client who had recommended her to me was wearing a classic bob, put there by me, and it was just that *look* that had attracted the new client to me. I got caught up in the semantics of the situation, not realizing her definition of what a *bob* haircut was, didn't extend to her friend's. What she saw her friend wearing wasn't a *bob* at all, but something *new* I had created.

So I layered it short and took out the volume below her occipital bone. She was devastated.

She had wanted what her friend had. When I tried to explain to her that what her friend was wearing was a *bob,* she adamantly insisted it was not; what *she* always got from the hairdresser was a bob, not what her friend had. It was too late at that point to explain to her that the bob was a general shape that lent itself to many lengths and looks; I had already screwed up.

I did my best to mollify her and gave her a refund and my abject apologies, but to no avail. I lost her forever as a client. And I had no one to blame but myself. I had broken a cardinal rule of communication: I had misread the client, and *assumed* we were on the same TV channel. I almost lost the original client as well. She was so disappointed at the result her friend had gotten, that she nearly quit coming to me as well, and it was a long time before she trusted me enough to send me any more of her friends. The circle one dissatisfied customer creates is every bit as wide as the one the stone makes when thrown into the pond. In our salon we estimate a regular client will contribute about five hundred dollars a year to our gross, through services and products purchased, and will send us an average of six acquaintances, who will do the same, and so on. The loss of one client is very costly and the damage to image is incalculable. It is hard to fix a dollar amount on that, unless you were to ask a salon owner who had gone bankrupt. He or she could probably give a fairly accurate estimate.

Misinterpreting what a client is telling you can be disastrous. Whenever you are in doubt as to whether or not a client really means what she is saying, continue to question her and lead the discussion until you are certain you are both *on the same page.* Sometimes, it may even be better to reschedule the appointment, should time dictate. It is better to lose a client because she was inconvenienced than to lose one who walked out with a style totally different from what she had anticipated.

Another consulting technique that is very effective, is brought to our attention by Thia Masciana of the International Hair Color Exchange. She says:

"Whenever you (stylist) are in doubt as to whether or not . . . you are hearing correctly what your client is saying, active listening skills can assist you in gaining more information. Novice psychologists are trained in a technique called reflective listening. Reflective listening can help you guide a client through the consultation so you get a clear picture of her expectations. This technique consists of listening to your client's statement about her hair and repeating part of what she says back to her. An example would sound like this: Your client says, 'I want a new look. This hair is boring.' You say, 'Boring?' She replies, 'Yes, I think I want it shorter.' To which you reply, 'Shorter?' She then expands on the idea of shorter and what that means to her. You can continue the reflective listening process throughout the conversation completing your sale by saying something like, 'So, what I'm hearing you say is, you would like to have your hair off your neck and directed back on the sides. Most of your ear will be exposed. That will really show off your eyes and cheekbones beautifully.'

"At the end of your conversation, both you and your client should have a clear word picture of what will take place.

"You may think this reflective listening technique sounds forced or funny. However, clients don't pick up on the fact that you are repeating part of what they have said back to them, they simply give you more information.

"From that information, you can deliver a product both you and your client will enjoy."

Learn to read body language also. There are several good texts on the subject. Your librarian or local bookstore should be able to help you choose a good text. There are the obvious tip-offs most of us are aware of that tell us what the person before us is really saying, such as folded arms and crossed legs implying the person isn't receptive at this time to our ideas, but there are hundreds more signals we give off and aren't conscious of that, once understood, can be invaluable tools in communicating with our clients.

Above all, look beyond what a person is saying and decipher what it is they are really after. Practice will improve how you read people and what is actually on their minds.

REVIEW

1. *Individuals sometimes don't communicate well, even with themselves:* By not fully understanding themselves, oftentimes a client cannot fully express what it is they are really after.

2. *Recognizing when what a person states verbally may not be what they mean:* If you suspect a dichotomy, look for what the client is really saying.

3. *Getting the client to communicate their real desires:* Be attentive to keys in what they are saying; i.e., when they show you a picture of a style they like, look for similar facial or other features they might share with the model.

CHAPTER 3

How to Establish Yourself as the Authority: Even if It's Your First Day Out of School

CHAPTER LEARNING OBJECTIVES

The stylist successfully mastering this chapter will know:

1. *How to structure the initial meeting with the client so that professional authority is established.*
2. *What the basis for that authority is and why each of us has it regardless of experience.*
3. *How to get the authority in the client-stylist relationship back where it belongs—in the hands of the stylist, even when the client has been controlling the situation.*
4. *Some of the reasons clients at times don't respect our judgement and what to do to change their attitude.*

Unless you establish yourself as the professional in the client-stylist relationship, you will be forever doomed to perform hair services at the client's whim. What that will mean is that you will sacrifice your creativity, your knowledge and craft, and ultimately your respect among both clients and fellow stylists. It will affect your pocketbook as well!

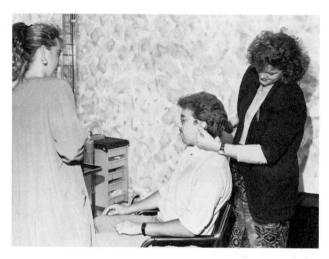

Fig. 3.1 Establish yourself as the professional—take charge.

If there were a list of Ten Commandments necessary to being a good hair stylist, at the top of the list would be, "Thou shalt never say to a client, 'Howdjawantyerhair?'!" That is absolutely the worst sin a stylist can ever commit, an even darker felony than giving a bad haircut. A bad haircut will grow out and the memory of it eventually fade. The client's impression of you if your first words to her are "howdjalikeyerhair?" will never die. Forever, you will be branded in her mind as unprofessional.

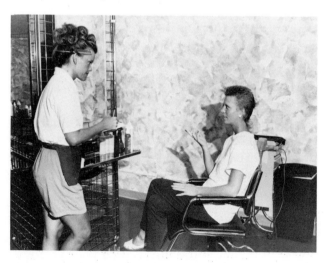

Fig. 3.2

Listen to the sound of those words: *How'd ya want yer hair done today?* Doesn't it sound like a waitress in a bad steak joint? Not to disparage waitresses—a good food service person with a professional manner in a quality establishment would never approach a diner with that question, but would probably say something like, "I'd like to suggest our leg of lamb today, Madam—it's superb." See the difference? One is a waitress, putting in hours in a menial job, whereas the second is a professional, with a career in food service. The second person will probably end up owning the restaurant.

First impression. An incomplete sentence gramatically, but a very complete one as far as importance. First impressions are many and various and include more that just the first time you physically meet and greet the client.

A first impression is made during initial phone contacts. A first impression is made when someone recommends you or your salon to the client. A first impression is made when a client views your advertisement in the newspaper, sees your billboard, or hears about you on the radio. A first impression is made when she walks into the salon. A first impression is made when she is greeted by the receptionist or anyone else in the salon.

First impressions are literally chains of impressions. When a client sits in your chair for the first time, she has already received many *first impressions.* That's why she's there. An impression somewhere along the way, or a series or combinations of impressions has convinced her that this is where she should be to get the thing she desires.

Most of those impressions will be good and positive or else she wouldn't be there, but there may be a negative one or two among the bunch. For instance, a good friend has raved about your work and so she made the appointment, but when she walked in, the receptionist was curt (as well as smoking a cigarette at the front desk). The social pressure to keep the appointment was strong enough that she didn't walk back out again, but that's why she's sitting there with negative body language—folded arms and legs.

Or, her experience in other salons may have been negative. Have you ever wondered why someone would go to the trouble of making an appointment with you only to arrive in almost a fighting mood? You know you haven't done anything to her—you only met her twenty seconds ago—so why is she so upset? It might be that you've inherited the legacy of a dozen bad experiences. Not fair, but that's life.

The point is, realize that the client didn't just arrive out of the blue. There were things that influenced her to come to you and the great majority of them were positive influences or else she would be somewhere else. Even if some of the impressions she's had already aren't positive, most of them were or she wouldn't be there.

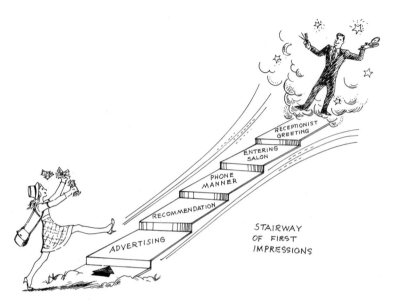

Fig. 3.3 There is more than one *first impression*.
There may be many, and they are all links
in the chain that brought the client to you,
or *steps* in the process. Make all of your
first impressions positive ones!

Use that knowledge to your benefit. Even if it's your first day out of school, and your state beauty license still smells new, realize that you still know more than your client does about doing hair. Do you think for a minute that if the client could do her hair better that a hairstylist she'd be spending money in salons? Not on your life!

Take charge of the situation at once. You should be the one to utter the first words, and those words should be designed to establish your authority in a nonthreatening manner.

Fledgling stylists and students often labor under the misconception that one must build up a lengthy period of time behind the chair before they will be qualified to perform an effective consultation. Nothing could be farther from the truth. Indeed, if you wait until you have the experience you think you need, you will probably be out of the business.

Being nervous is all right. There's nothing wrong with you, provided you don't let those nerves keep you from doing your job. Remember, when you go out to meet that first client, that even though you may be young in the busi-

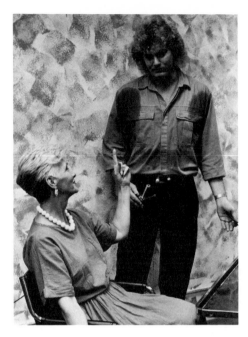

Fig. 3.4 Never let them see you sweat.

ness, you have infinitely more knowledge about hair and styling that virtually all clients do.

Good consultation techniques will help build a clientele faster that any other means. It beats advertising hands down, if only because although a good ad will get someone in the door one time, a good consultation will get them back again and again.

Properly structured, the consultation period achieves many things. It will establish even the newest stylist as a solid professional in the eyes of the client and create in the client the impression that this is the best stylist possible for her particular wants and needs.

To make efficient use of time, the consultation should take from five to fifteen minutes, at the end of which the client and stylist should be in agreement on the service and desired result, with a clear mental picture of what that will be.

A successful consultation will satisfy these goals:

1. It will establish the stylist as the *professional.*
2. It will give the client the confidence that what she is to receive is what she wants and needs.

31

3. It will leave the client secure that she will leave the salon satisfied, but knowing that this is not the end, that her needs will change in time, and that this is the stylist who can effect that change when the time comes.
4. It will give the stylist a clear picture of what the client wants and needs.

It sounds very easy to those of us who are experienced, but to the neophyte just the idea of leading a client in a discussion about her hair can create a severe case of stage fright. Just realize that those fears are related mostly to lack of experience and not to lack of *ability.*

The new stylist, especially, needs to realize that control in a consulting situation is established at the very beginning. *She* takes charge by going up to the client and introducing herself professionally, which includes a handshake, even with another woman.

"Why, good morning, Mrs. Future! It's so nice to meet you. I understand Sally Present recommended me to you. Let me promise you that I'll do my very best to give you the look you want. Please come with me to my styling area so that we can discuss your hair."

Then, *lead* the client to the consulting area and indicate where the client should sit.

Although there is no one right way to conduct a consultation, there are many wrong ways. A detailed analysis of consultations is provided in Chapter Four, "How to Structure the Consultation."

Be certain to offer your hand in a professional manner. Just a few years back, there was some debate about when to shake a woman's hand, and there was

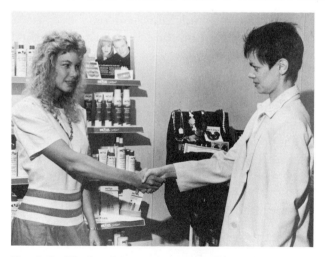

Fig. 3.5 The handshake is the symbol of today's businesswoman and businessman.

even more debate about if and when women should shake each other's hands. The etiquette has completely changed in the past few years, as women have achieved more and more parity in the workplace, and it is commonly accepted that in matters of protocol, such as the business handshake, women are on the same page as men. There is probably still a debate over this etiquette, but as far as hairstylists (and other professionals) are concerned, don't get too involved in such arguments as whether or not a woman should remain seated while shaking hands, or should a man only shake a woman's hand when she offers it. Those rules are stale and dated and don't apply in today's business settings. In business situations, people shake hands. The one in authority is the one who offers his or her hand first. Watch a good salesperson. He or she will leap to be the first to offer his or her hand. It puts that person in control immediately.

Just the act of you offering your hand to the client first does much of the work in establishing your professionalism and in establishing control of the situation. Offering your hand as you begin to introduce yourself locks yourself into the client's mind as someone in charge and it is a powerful tool in setting the whole tone of the subsequent proceedings.

Lead the client to wherever you'll be consulting and direct her to where she should sit. Never take for granted that people know what you want them to do, at least the first visit. A person entering a salon for the first time literally doesn't know which of the seventeen chairs in the waiting area she is permitted to sit in and will hesitate before picking one unless the receptionist is well-trained enough to direct her to a specific chair after greeting her.

I have a personal preference when greeting a first-time client. I like to walk up to her, shake her hand and greet her, and then sit down with her in the reception area, of course, indicating a seat for her. I have established control by doing so, but have also made the situation a little less threatening for her by beginning our conversation in a casual atmosphere. I spend just a minute thanking her for coming in as in the above example with "Mrs. Future," and spend a minute or two in genial conversation, perhaps touching on the mutual friend that referred her to me, saying something complimentary about her. Then, I rise and ask her to accompany me back to the styling and consultation area.

The reason I do this is that I've observed stylist's greeting techniques, and it is common to see a stylist greet a new client with a "Hi ya, Mrs. Whoever, follow me," and trot off to some area at the back of the salon, while Mrs. Whoever runs behind in her high heels, trying not to trip and lose sight of the vanishing stylist. Just a minute or so spent thusly in the reception area, helps take the edge off what probably is a terrifying moment for the new client, *the first time at a new salon,* and helps get her in a receptive frame of mind that will be warmer to your subsequent suggestions than if you'd just won a foot-race to your chair with her.

I'd like to claim credit for figuring out this technique by myself, but I owe the credit to one of the best food servers I've ever seen. She worked at one of the finer New Orleans restaurants I frequented, and I used to watch her in amazement. She was a marvel. She took care of twice as many tables as any of the other servers, but never seemed harried or hurried. She also made twice as much money!

She had a trick of hesitating with the new arrival before she seated them, passing back and forth a bit of jovial banter, and she made the pause seem like she had all the time in the world, when she was, in fact, the busiest person in the place. Then, upon the patron's departure, she did the same thing, pausing just a few seconds to exchange pleasantries. The result was that the diner felt relaxed during the entire dining experience, tipped her well, and asked for her table the next visit. As a matter of fact, *all* of the diners at her tables were what she referred to as "call customers," persons who had requested her area.

She would have been a huge success in any line she chose. Even though she had more to do than the other servers, she also sold the most *extras*. When the other servers got behind, they omitted to ask the diners present if they wanted a piece of pie or a dish of sherbert. Not my wizard waitress! "You've got to have some of the Bananas Foster," she'd say, and the diner, groaning, would force himself to stuff a few more mouthfuls of dessert into his or her mouth. The funny thing was, even though she sold more such extras and took care of more diners and more tables, she never made anyone feel hurried or that they were occupying a seat that was needed for the next diner, and yet her tables turned over quicker than anyone else's.

She should have been a consultant to the hairstyling business.

When you come across a person who deals well with the public such as my friend in New Orleans, study him or her and what they are doing. They will have important lessons to impart that you can use in your own line of work.

Getting back to our own clients, after you've made them feel comfortable and welcome by offering her refreshment, drop the small talk and ease into the consultation. This may be difficult to do, especially for newer stylists, who may have been dreading that supposed *awful moment* when they have to actu-ally suggest something to the client and then do it. Keep on course, stay with the program, and don't be too chatty, and the client will realize that you are a businesslike person and respond in kind.

We've already established that it's bad form to ask the client "Howdja-wantyerhairdone?" Let's assume no one is ever going to do that again (if they have been), and won't start if they haven't. There is another extreme and that is the hairdresser who seats the client and then imperiously announces, "You need a bob. That's what I'm going to give you," or something to that effect. This approach may work with some, but with many others, those are fighting words and the client may get right up out of the chair and thrust her jaw at you and respond with something like, "And who died and appointed *you* President?" Not the words you want whispered in your ear, I presume!

The approach we use in our salon goes something like this:

"Marilyn, because this is the first time we have met, this presents a unique situation for me. As of now, I don't know any of your likes and dislikes, prejudices and preferences. Therefore, before you tell me any of those, I'd like a few minutes to look over your hair and features and ask you a few related questions, and then I'd like to suggest what I feel would look best on you and be the easiest for you to maintain."

At this point, I also interject an example to illustrate why I want to do this.

"The reason I want to do it this way, is that knowing your likes and dislikes can restrict my creative input. For example, if you would happen to be an artist and I went up to you and said, 'Marilyn, I'd like you to paint me a picture, but just don't put any oak trees in it.' Well, from that point on, all you'd probably see *are* oak trees! It's the same with your hair. You may say something like, 'Do anything you like, Les, but leave my length,' thinking you're giving me virtual *carte blanche,* but, in effect, closing me off, creatively.

"When I finish my analysis, I'll tell you what I think we should do, and you can do one of three things (1) tell me my idea is great—let's do it; (2) my idea is terrible—let's don't; or, (3) part of my idea is good but not all of it. If you chose either of the latter, at least we have a basis for communication, and you may well like my suggestion well enough to want to try that."

That sounds rather long-winded, but in practice it cuts down the consultation time considerably. The great majority of time, the client says, "I like that idea. Let's go for it." Even at the times when they disagree, the basis for communicating is set and she realizes that I truly am a professional and that I know something about hairstyling. She also knows by the way I presented myself that I'm not trying to shove my ideas down her throat and that I respect her own opinion. Usually, I'll say as an aside, before I begin my analysis, that "Whatever I suggest to you, Marilyn, is just that—a *suggestion*. I'll give you the reasons I think we should do whatever I suggest, but the only opinion that counts is yours, and whatever we do will be your decision."

When you approach a client in this fashion, you will be doing several positive things that reinforce you as the authority. You've let them know that *yes,* you do have definite ideas as to what will work and why, but that also you respect her wishes and opinions as well, and that it is her opinion that will win out should there be a conflict. This takes any threatening aspects of the consultation out of the situation and leaves the client assured that she is in competent hands.

Clients are dying to have a hairdresser tell them what looks good on them—they're just particular about the way the hairdresser goes about doing so.

Those of you who have been hairdressers and stylists for very long have run into countless clients who have mused and said to you, "I wish I could go to (New York, Chicago, Los Angeles, pick any other city bigger than the one you're in) and have (current TV hairstyling celebrity) do my hair and tell me how I should wear it."

I thought when I left Lakeville, Indiana (population 1,117) to go to South Bend, Indiana (population 168,000), I would cease to hear that. Then, I thought those words were history when I moved to Indianapolis. When I moved to New Orleans, I was sure they would never be heard again, but sure enough I heard them again. It was the same when I worked in Chicago and Los Angeles. It was the same *everywhere!* I heard it in salons that were imminently famous, and I heard it in salons whose name had not been heard of in the next town.

People very desperately *want* a stylist who is strong enough to suggest a style for them. Many clients are sick and tired of going to stylists who say, "Howdjawantyerhairdone?" They *yearn* for someone to take control and tell them what's best for them (provided it's done in a nonthreatening, diplomatic, *professional* fashion).

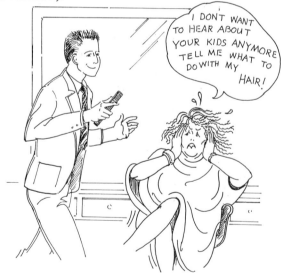

Fig. 3.6

If you will use this approach with your clients beginning today, you will be amazed at the difference in the way your clients begin treating you and how quickly the word gets out that there's a terrific new stylist in town (even if you've been at the same pop stand for twenty years!).

For those who *have* been working with the same clientele for a long time—don't be afraid to change your presentation. No one will laugh at you or think you've slipped a cog, if, instead of saying, "Hi, Beverly, cut it like the last twenty-seven times?", you try the above approach.

Here's a good way to begin if you've slipped into some bad habits. Begin booking an extra fifteen minutes with that longtime client, and when she arrives, say something to her like, "Say, Beverly, I got to thinking the other night about how long I've been doing your hair, and I'm ashamed because I realize I might have been taking you for granted. I value you highly as a friend and client and starting right now, I want to take steps to ensure that I'll never take you for granted again. I thought of a new look that would look great on you. Will you let me explain it? If you decide you'd rather not change, that's fine, but I'd like to go over my ideas with you and tell you why I think it would look good."

Even if she has you do her hair the same way you have been doing it, you've raised her consciousness of you and impressed her that you are concerned with her well-being and are a professional as well.

Stylists who have started doing this with their older clients tell me that several of them confided to them that they were just about ready to switch stylists, thinking they were going to go to their graves with the same ten-year-old style. When the looks you're creating look as if they might belong in the Smithsonian, it's time to reevaluate your client-stylist relationships!

It's a good idea to mark out extra time every fifth or sixth time you service the same client and do another consultation with them. It makes them feel appreciated and think that if they are ever going to get a new look, that you're the one who can provide it for them.

During the first time I do a new person's hair, I plant a seed in their mind, that I believe keeps them coming back to me, especially when they are desirous of a change.

I say, "Mrs. Future, I firmly believe a woman should change her hairstyle occasionally, at least once a year. Now, that doesn't necessarily mean a *drastic* change, it can be as subtle as changing where you part your hair." Paint your words with analogies. "Mrs. Future, it's like that green couch in your living room. Every week, you move it and clean behind it and under it, but you always put it back in exactly the same place. After awhile, it becomes invisible. The same thing happens with our appearance. Wearing the same style too long

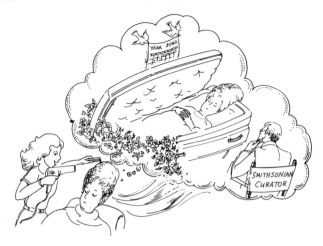

Fig. 3.7

makes us invisible to those in our lives we don't want to be invisible to. A change, even a slight change is desirable occasionally. It's with that philosophy that from time to time, I'll suggest something different for you. Is that okay with you?"

I can count on my fingers the times clients have said they'd rather I didn't, that they'd like to keep the same style until they turned room temperature.

We keep file cards on our clients with all kinds of interesting information (except dates of birth—we don't dare do that!). Many times, I'll say to the client, after the above spiel, "You know that file card you helped fill out Mrs. Future? Well, on it I always enter exactly how I cut your hair, so that not only myself but also anyone else in the salon can duplicate the cut should I happen to be sick when you need it done, but what I never do is record how I dried or dressed it. I do that for a specific reason. I feel very strongly that a woman should change her appearance as I've said, and, from time to time I'll suggest a new look to you. If you want to continue with the same cut, I can always duplicate that by just glancing at your card, but I *won't remember exactly how I styled it the last time, so for one day at least you'll probably get a slightly different look.* I do that on purpose. If you like it, great, but if you don't like it as well, nothing is lost, because the cut is the same and the first time you dry it yourself you can do it the same way. Nothing has been changed, except temporarily. I'm telling you this up front for the reasons I've said. Do you mind?"

No one, not *one single person* has ever said to me after that, "No, no, don't do that; please write down exactly the way you dry it!" Never. People *want* to change. They just want the change to come about in a nonthreatening, safe way.

You be the professional and the authority; don't concede it to the client!

REVIEW

1. *Structure the initial meeting to establish professional authority:* Remember that first impressions are many. Do everything in your power to ensure that *all* the client's first impressions are positive, from phone contact to the first step she makes inside the salon. Take charge of the consultation immediately by offering your hand, introducing yourself, and directing the client where to sit. Simply take charge, but do it in a nonthreatening, friendly manner.

2. *Your basis for authority:* No matter how many times the client has had her hair done and no matter if your license still has wet print on it, you *still* know more about hair than she ever will.

3. *How to regain lost authority:* Start off with the old client (book extra time) by apologizing for taking her for granted and tell her you'd like to suggest a new look for her, and this is why you think she'd like it. Always offer concrete reasons, don't just say you "think" it "might" look better.

4. *Why clients don't respect our judgement and how you can change their attitude:* Clients have been exposed to too many "Howdjawantyerhairdones?" They look upon many hairdressers as unprofessional. Treat them in a professional manner in the ways suggested and the attitude will never form in new clients and disappear in old ones.

Take Charge!

CHAPTER 4

How to Structure the Consultation

CHAPTER LEARNING OBJECTIVES

The stylist successfully mastering this chapter will know:

1. *The proper physical layout of the consulting area.*
2. *The psychology behind a successful consultation.*
3. *Understanding what the client is after.*
4. *Timing the consultation.*
5. *Conducting the consultation in the direction you want it to go.*
6. *Understanding that the consultation doesn't end when you begin to cut hair.*

Before you even begin your first consultation, it would be advantageous to determine the best possible physical layout in which to conduct the consultation. With some salons, this may be very limited, because of prior design and space requirements, but if at all possible, a quiet, private space might be provided.

Although you and I are accustomed to discussing coloring, perming, and cutting theories and ideas freely, many clients are sensitive about having their hair discussed in front of others, or where others might overhear—especially other clients of the opposite sex.

Be doubly conscious of possible sensitivity when discussing coloring techniques or ideas with a client, as a great many people want to keep the fact that

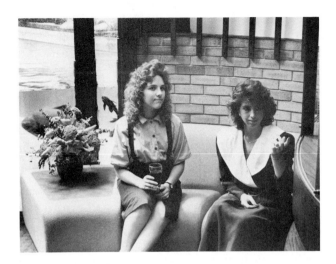

Fig. 4.1 If possible, prepare a quiet, private consulting area.

they cover their gray hair a secret. Nothing is more mortifying (and more likely to drive a client away) than to have a stylist declare to the world that "your hair is about sixty percent gray—let's cover it with Number 6 Wonderbar Color!" Even when everyone in the world knows she tints her hair, and she knows they know it—she won't want it broadcast. Trust me on this!

Spend a few minutes thinking about your consulting style to see if perhaps you haven't become desensitized in this area. It's easy to do—we spend all day,

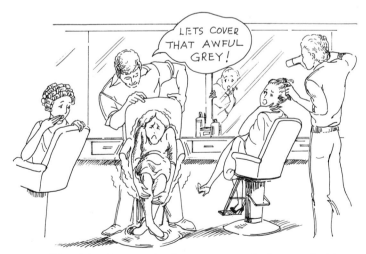

Fig. 4.2 Communication systems: *tele*phone, *tele*vision, *tele*stylist!

41

five days a week, talking about hair, hair, hair—and after awhile, discussing hair becomes as natural and as necessary as breathing. We tend to forget that the client doesn't do this and regards her hair in a more personal way.

If you are a salon owner, observe your staff and be sure they are being circumspect in their conversations with their clientele. You may want to make this a topic at your next salon meeting and solicit ideas on how to make your consultations more private and professional, if they have developed a town meeting atmosphere.

As always, in every phase of your dealings with your clients, try and put yourself in their place and imagine your emotions should someone treat you the way you treat them. It is a good idea to step back every so often and reevaluate procedures, not only in consultations but other areas of the client-stylist relationship as well.

In one of the salons I owned years ago, we had a system where none of the stylists got their hair cut in our own salon. When a haircut was needed by one of the stylists, they would go to another salon where they were not known.

They would not tell the stylist cutting their hair that they were also a stylist, but would pretend to be something else, a nurse, a plumber, a housewife, a secretary, so as not to receive the special treatment they would probably receive if the stylist realized they were a fellow professional.

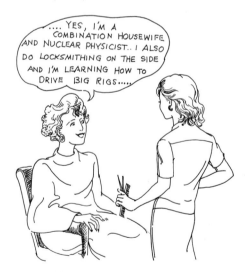

Fig. 4.3 Visit other salons, *incognito,* and see what you enjoy about the salon and then incorporate it into your own.

As soon as they left the salon and went to their car, they would immediately write down five things they liked about the experience, and *five things they didn't like*. Then, at our monthly salon meeting, each stylist would share her list with the rest of us. Going into a salon purely as a client will open one's eyes and make you see things from a different point of view. We all started to realize that many of the things we disliked about our visit to the other salon were things we, ourselves, were doing! The experience made each of us much more aware of how we were treating our own clients. On the other side of the coin, we picked up many useful ideas about how to make the client feel even more comfortable and welcome, and incorporated those ideas into our own philosophy.

You might try this idea occasionally. When you need a trim, instead of getting the stylist who works next to you to cut it, make an appointment at another salon and pay close attention to what you like and what you dislike about the whole procedure, from the moment you make the appointment over the phone to when you pay your final bill. The relatively small amount you pay for a hair service will return itself tenfold in the new understandings you'll come away with.

If total privacy cannot be achieved in your present salon setting, if the salon is somewhat crowded with stations clustered near one another, be careful to keep your voice level low enough that others can't eavesdrop on your conversation with the client.

If you are fortunate in having some latitude in designing a consulting room, there are several basics that should be considered. First, there should be a mirror so that the client might see herself, which will aid in communicating. Seating, of course, should be comfortable. There is a well-known theory that if you want to be in charge, *your* chair, should you use one in this stage, should be higher than the clients, but this theory you may or may not subscribe to.

If you are planning a new salon or redesigning the present one to include a consulting room, you might want to allow for a television and VCR or even one of the computer simulators that show a client what certain styles or color or perm effects would look like on them. Usually, such an investment would prove to be a wise one.

In our own salon, we haven't yet added the computer simulator, but we do utilize video by preparing our own introduction tape, which is shown to the new client. In it, we give a short fifteen-minute discussion in which we explain our salon philosophy; briefly explain the services we offer; and introduce staff members and specialists, such as our masseuse, skin care and makeup technician, body wrap technician, colorist, perm technician, and so on. We leave the client alone in the room with the tape and some refreshment, and when the tape is over, we come back in and begin our consultation. (We also make sure to reenter quickly after the tape ends so that the client doesn't have to sit there with the TV broadcasting snow!)

We don't experience much difficulty in having the client take this extra time, as we are viewed by the public as being an upscale salon, and new clients more or less expect to spend more time with us. We also prepare the new client for this portion by having the salon coordinator (receptionist) explain to her over the phone that extra time is scheduled for her first visit so that we might better serve her needs.

In another type of salon, this may not be feasible; however, don't dismiss the idea entirely, as styling time isn't lost. Schedule the new client so that she is viewing the tape while you are working on the preceding client, thereby saving you time when you enter into the one-on-one portion of your consultation.

If there are no options other than to use the styling station itself, it is still important, and perhaps doubly so, to prepare your station properly. It should be immaculate, which should go without saying, and uncluttered. The mirror and all appurtenances should be spotless. Hair care products that might be out should be closed and not have old gel or mousse or product dripping from them. In other words, it should appear the same way you would want it to should you know the beauty inspector were to show up for an inspection. A clean, neat area presents a strong, positive, *professional* impression to the new (and old) client and demonstrates that you have respect for yourself, your work, and her as well. You exhibit a professional who respects her equipment and clientele.

Providing the right setting and atmosphere is critical. A clean, uncluttered setting creates one impression; a messy one, another. Pictures of the kiddies; macramé hanging from the walls; old, dated hairstyle photos that belong in the Smithsonian; brushes strangled with hair from previous brushings; a sterilizer with debris floating freely in it, all create an unprofessional, amateurish effect in the client's mind. Not to mention rendering them nauseous, perhaps. Picture your doctor's, lawyer's, or accountant's office, and use them for models. Everyone is undoubtedly aware that you are proud of your kids, but the business office is not the place to display their gap-toothed smiles. Nor should examples of award-winning macramé or knitting nor cutesy stuffed animals or buttons with clever sayings be displayed. The scene presented should be clean, neat, and professional.

An effective consultation has a certain psychology behind it. Before you ever meet and greet the client, picture in your mind the result you want. You will want the interview to fit within a certain time span, say ten or fifteen minutes, and you will want to always be in control and to direct the consultation in the

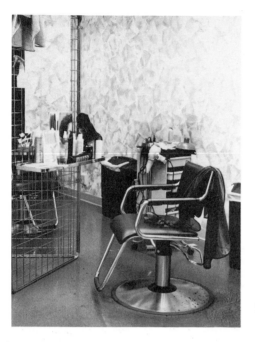

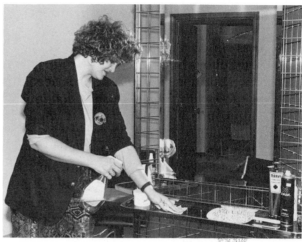

Fig. 4.4 Your styling area imparts a powerful message to the client.

proper direction and not meander off in irrelevant discussions that have nothing to do with the purpose in mind.

Taking charge immediately of the consultation stamps you as the person in charge to the client and gives you the aura of being the professional. Preambling your opening remarks to the client as some of the examples in Chapter Three will help establish your authority and set the tone for the rest of the consultation.

An important rule to follow during the consultation is to remember not to offer too many styling suggestions to the client. When you give more than two or three options, the client becomes confused and can't make up her mind, and the consultation can drag on forever with no decision being made, or at best, an unsure one. Too many choices almost always will be detrimental to your goal, that of guiding the client to the best look you are able to provide. For instance, when you are making suggestions and using pictures to give her an idea of what it is you have in mind, don't show her more than two or three examples of different looks. Looking at seven or eight (or more!) pictures of beautiful models, all with different styles, is akin to letting a small child run amok in a candy store—they can't make up their mind! The client will want everything, and just as she seems to make up her mind on one look, another will begin to look more attractive, and then you're off to the races.

Halfway through the cut, she'll have a change of heart and decide that she would rather have the style on page 37 than the one on page 12 you thought she'd settled on.

Also, when using pictures as an example, don't oversell the final effect. Don't lead her to believe that she'll look just like the girl in the photo, but instead get across to her that the example shown is just that, an example, and that even though it will be cut and styled the same way, it won't look exactly the same on her, but will be individualized for her because of the differences between her and the subject of the photo.

A good technique is to have the client place her hand over the face of the model shown, leaving just the hairstyle visible and tell her to imagine that style on her own head. When we look at photos, sometimes we fail to realize all that has gone into the picture. The stylist who has done the style has selected the best possible model and has spent a great deal of time preparing the hair. The subject has been photographed with the best possible professional lighting techniques with the most favorable makeup effects. The end result is a combination of many factors that cannot be duplicated in a normal salon setting. Make the client aware of that in a diplomatic way, meaning, don't tell her the model in the photograph is gorgeous and she more closely resembles a lower number on the one-to-ten scale!

Know what the average client is after. And what is that? Simple—she just wants to be the most gorgeous, beautiful, sexy woman imaginable—or, at least, within her limitations. Most of us are like that—we want to look attractive not only to ourselves, but also to others. Assume this is the goal of your client and very seldom will you be in error. You don't even have to come out and say this; in fact, many times if you do, you'll receive a denial. The client will say, "Oh, I'm way beyond that—I'm too old," or something similar, but it's difficult to imagine someone who doesn't want to appear more desirable to someone else. And if they don't, chances are they aren't sitting in a stylist's chair. They're not clients of anyone, usually, or if they are, all they want is to get their hair chopped off so they fit loosely within the parameters of what society accepts.

They are not the norm. They are not the clients upon which to build a successful clientele.

Time is money. Therefore, the consultation should have a time requirement. Normally, this procedure should take no more than ten to twenty minutes, at the outside. With the tightness of this requirement, it is important that you stick to a discussion of the hair and style itself, and guide the client in the proper direction, keeping the consultation train on the track and from wandering very far afield.

Establish yourself as the professional, the one in charge, using the suggested openings or one of your own, and plunge directly into your diagnosis. Tell her you believe she should allow you to do ___ to her hair, and give her the reason she should let you do this. Tell her the benefits (for her) of following your advice and give her the best mental picture of what she will look like that you are capable of, remembering to always strive to be on the same TV channel. When you are done with this part of the presentation, ask her if she thinks you should do this. Phrase this so that a "yes" answer is easiest. Try to phrase all leading questions so that it is easier to answer with an affirmative reply.

The consultation is a sales pitch. You are selling a client a hairstyle. Your entire job as a stylist is in sales, in every single aspect. I hate to hear stylists say, "Oh, I'm not a salesperson—I'm a *stylist,*" as if there were something degrading about selling someone something, or that they're some sort of great artist, pure and above the commonality that they view sales to be. If you're not into sales and have an antipathy toward sales, I would daresay you're not going to last long in the business; if you do, you're not going to be highly successful at it. If you should happen to view salesmanship in a negative fashion, you might do well to reevaluate your opinion if you expect to do very well in this profession.

Successful selling is very simple. You make a presentation, after gauging the client's needs and wants, and you ask for the sale. You ask for the sale as quickly as you can, expecting a *yes* answer. You structure the sale question in such a way as to make it easier for the client to say *yes* than to say *no.*

Here are two examples of the right and wrong way to ask for the sale:

1. Wrong way: "So, Mrs. Future, which of the four looks I've described to you would you like to have me do?"
2. Right way: "Mrs. Future, this is the style that I recommend. Don't you agree that we should cut it this way?"

In the first example, you've left the possibilities too open-ended. She's liable to say, "Well, uh, gee, I don't know. Can we look behind door number three again?"

If you've structured the consultation properly so far, and then asked for the sale and the client doesn't buy, what you've encountered is known as an *objection,* in sales parlance. That's all right; all salespeople meet objections. The good ones overcome them, and as quickly and efficiently as possible. Determine what her *real* objection is. Is it that she views the proposed style as not being attractive on her; does she think it will be too hard to maintain; or is she under the impression she will have to purchase a lot of costly products to maintain the style properly? If you think you know her objection, counter it immediately and then ask for the sale again.

"Mrs. Future, I know you think this style will take a lot of work. It actually requires less work than you think, and I'll show you a very easy way to maintain it that only takes ten minutes from start to finish. I promise you that you'll be able to do what I'll show you before you leave today. That's the best thing about this style that makes it better than what you're wearing now—the ease of maintenance will give you a lot more freedom from care. May I shampoo you and prep your hair so that we can start?"

Sometimes the objection voiced is not the real objection. Keep looking for the real objection, but don't become argumentative. If the client is really stubborn about your choice, back off and offer another idea. But don't be fearful of objections. They are a normal and expected part of sales. After each objection encountered, meet it, offer a reason why she should buy (your idea), and ask for the sale.

Once she has said *yes,* stop selling! This is very important. Many of us are unsure about what we are selling and we tend to oversell. I have seen many stylists convince the client to try the look they are proposing and then talk the client right out of it by overselling it. They talk nonstop on the way to the shampoo area, during the shampoo, and on the way back about the virtues of the choice the client has made, and in so doing, have caused themselves to appear insecure. This is when the client begins to have second thoughts and starts to cross her legs and fold her arms and get a glinty look in her eye. Even if she allows you to perform the style at this point, she is probably going to be disappointed, for no style every created will be able to give her everything you've promised. Her expectation will far outstrip the reality.

After you've made the sale (she's said *yes* to your suggestion), congratulate her on her smart decision and tell her how much she's going to like it, and then shut up!

"Mrs. Future, you've done a nice thing for yourself in deciding to go with this style. You're going to be very pleased at how easy it is to maintain and delighted at how much your husband is going to like the new you."

Then, get onto the next phase in the consultation process, which is to begin preparing her for future sales, which we'll get into later on in the chapter.

There are many techniques that are valuable to know when you are selling someone an idea or a product. For example, when you ask for the sale, phrasing your question so that it more easily elicits an affirmative response, you can even nod your head up and down slightly as you pose the question. This is a subliminal tactic that is done subtly, but it works. This, and other such tactics may sound underhanded, but they are recognized sales techniques, and because you are advising the client in a professional way, and backing up your advice with your expertise and knowledge, you are doing nothing more than any other professional person. As long as you believe in the validity of your proposal (and I hope you do!), there is nothing wrong with nudging the client into the direction you know she should go.

It's a competitive world, like it or not, and if you practice being passive, someone out there will eat your lunch. We may want to think of ourselves as some sort of pure artist, but the fact is that although you may be the greatest hairstylist in the world, unless you have clientele coming in the door to practice your art, you are, in effect, an artist without a portfolio (and driving an older car than you would probably want, too). Aggressiveness in business is the keynote today, and very necessary to remain in business.

It is not a bad idea to attend as many general sales technique classes as you do hair design classes. This is really and truly a sales and marketing business we find ourselves in—the product we market is our ability to design hair. General Motors may feel very honestly that they have one of the best cars manufactured, but they don't sit around in the executive suite with a prima donna complex, sucking on a bottle of Perrier, saying, ''We're the best so we don't have to lower ourselves telling people that. People will just recognize our quality and flock to our showrooms on their own.'' The success stories in life, from General Motors and Coca-Cola down to the hottest salon in your area, not only put out a quality product, but they also tell people about it—over and over. They spend tons of money instructing and educating their salespeople in how to sell more effectively, and part of that strategy is to make it easy for the client to say *yes* to the question you seek a *yes* answer to.

If you have friends who are in other, traditional sales fields, such as life insurance, home party plans, car sales, or executive recruiting, ask them if you can attend their sales meetings. If not, ask them for any books or materials they would recommend that give good sales techniques. Read motivational books and listen to inspirational tapes. Spend as much time, if not more, on learning good sales techniques as you do on the technical side of your craft. One cannot work without the other, although a disproportionate amount of time is usually spent on the technical side, and not nearly enough on the sales side.

When the client agrees to your idea, begin the proposed service immediately. Once you are into the service, it is okay to reinforce the sale as long as you don't overdo it. Harken to the Bard's words, ''Methinks he doth protest too much!'' If you make a relatively simple hairstyle into the eighth wonder of the world, the reality, when presented, won't satisfy the expectations, and you'll end up with a dissatisfied client. Don't sell a permanent wave to client and then tell her story after story of clients of yours who've kept their waves for six

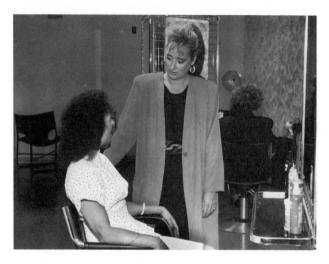

Fig. 4.5 Don't oversell the hair service.

or seven months before they needed another one. When she needs another one in three months, she won't remember that you told her those seven-month perm clients were the exception and that *maybe* hers would last as long; she'll remember them as being represented as the *norm* and then think she got a bad perm and that you owe her a redo. Tell her what the service will do *and no more.*

Sometimes you run into a tough client who puts up objection after objection. No matter what you suggest, she's negative toward the idea. A successful tactic, when that situation arises, is to make your next suggestion, give your reasons, and then zip your lip. Let silence work for you. Most of us are uncomfortable with silence. Sooner or later (usually sooner), she will say something, perhaps ask a question about your suggestion, and you can close the sale by answering the question succinctly and then asking for the sale again. "Don't you agree that this is what we should do?"

If it doesn't work the first time, use the tactic again. It will quickly dawn on her that these uncomfortable silences aren't going to end unless she's the one to end them, and usually she'll acquiesce to the sale.

When all else fails and none of your suggestions has met with approval, to avoid any more unnecessary time delays, simply ask her what she has in mind. If she tells you, fine, as long as you agree and don't think it will be a disaster. Then, go ahead and do it. If she has no idea at all, but still doesn't like any of your ideas, you can then do one of two things. You can go back to the idea you were most comfortable with and tell her again why you think this is what you should do and why, and ask for the sale again. Or, you can be honest with her and state that perhaps you aren't the stylist for her and that she may want to consult with someone else, perhaps in your own salon or at a salon you could recommend. I'm serious about this. There are no laws in any state I'm aware of that say you must sell something to every single prospect. Sometimes you're better off (and so is the client) by suggesting she go somewhere else.

Now, you don't want to get into the practice of chasing clients out of your salon; it's too hard to get them there in the first place! Do it very often and you won't have a business to speak of, but there are times when you have to have some integrity.

The looks and quality of service that leave your salon are a direct reflection upon *you,* and if those looks are not your best work and reflect the philosophy of your salon, then you are doing yourself a disservice. Each and every one of your clients is an advertisement for you. Determine what kind of advertising you want others to see.

We have an ironclad rule in our salon that clients are never to leave without their hair being styled and finished. They never leave with a wet head of hair, unless the look we are designing is a *wet look.* This may not fit your philosophy and doesn't mean our salon is *right* and yours is wrong—it is simply what is right for us. I have had clients who have said, "Look, I'm going right home and into the swimming pool. In ten minutes my hair will be wet again." My rejoinder to this is, "I understand, and you're right. All this work will disappear shortly. *But,* when you leave the salon, someone will see you and not know those circumstances and think that this is the way we style hair. You will be a bad advertisement for us, even if it's for only ten minutes, and we really don't want bad advertisements." Most of our clients understand this and comply. The ones that don't, we don't feel we can afford, because of the image they present for us.

I can't see any difference in the client who wishes to leave with her hair wet and unstyled, than the person of yesteryear who went to the market with rollers in her hair. Granted, it was only for a short trip to pick up milk and eggs, but how many times have you heard others laugh at the sight? Most of us agree that it is a very unattractive look to display in public and I can't see any difference between appearing in rollers at the supermarket and appearing in wet, messy hair coming out of our salon.

Once, I owned a salon in a racquetball club, and one of our "walls" was the Plexiglass partition that separated us from the giant whirlpool. We had many clients who had their hair cut and styled and left the salon to take twenty steps to the whirlpool where they would immerse their head. We still insisted on drying and styling their hair. You may see this as unreasonable, but we didn't feel that way at all. For twenty steps, that client was an advertisement. The result of our policy was that most people admired our integrity and became clients, partly because of the respect we demanded for our work. We enjoyed a full booking, had an overflow business with zero advertising, and were booked several weeks in advance. I closed the business when I decided to move out of state and another stylist re-opened it a few years later, in the same location. That stylist was every bit as talented as I perhaps am, and perhaps even more so, but has struggled from the very beginning, and I am convinced that at least part of the reason is due to relaxing of the rule we had, and allowing people to leave the salon with wet hair.

At any rate, it is important to not only have a philosophy toward your business, but to have it in more than name only. When you begin compromising what you believe in, whatever it is, you begin to lose the respect of not only clients but yourself as well.

Back to the obstinate client who insists you do something truly hideous, and you try to convince her otherwise, but end up doing what she wants; what will happen is this: When her best friend asks her who did her style, she won't say, "Well, I *made* Les do it, even though he wanted to do something else." No, she'll answer by saying, "Les". That's all. As far as anyone else knows, you tied her down and forced her into the look she's sporting.

Therefore, know the boundaries of style and fashion you respect, and when push comes to shove as it will occasionally, then don't cross the line. You'll not only maintain your own self-respect, but gain the respect of others, especially if it's done in a tactful manner.

Remember also, that style and fashion are arbitrary and a matter of personal taste. No one has appointed any stylist the Supreme Being and decreed that his or her taste is the only acceptable one, and in the final analysis, the only important opinion is that of the client. She's the one who's going to be wearing your creation, not you. She's the one who has to like it and feel at ease with it. She's the one who's going to have that inner glow because she feels good about her appearance, or feels like all eyes are on her critically, because her look is wrong for her. When it comes to differences of opinion about what anyone should wear, the only opinion that truly counts is the feeling of the one who will be wearing it. Respect her opinion as much as you would have her respect yours and never be derogatory in tone or manner, but assure her that while you disagree, you respect her thoughts and will do your best to deliver her into hands that will do what she desires, skillfully and cheerfully. When that happens, if it's performed correctly, then you may have lost a client but you will have lost none of her respect and she'll speak highly of you to others.

Assuming this doesn't happen but once every ten years or so, and that most clients will follow your lead and let you do what you prescribe, and the result turns out every bit as wonderfully as you predicted, then don't assume the consultation is over. Consultations are not a one-time affair, performed at the beginning of the first service. Consulting with the client should be an ongoing procedure as long as you are maintaining a client-stylist relationship and as long as you are servicing her hair needs.

Each time she comes back in, you should be ready with suggestions for her. This doesn't by any means involve suggesting major design changes for her each time, but something should be suggested each and every time she comes in that wasn't the visit before. Get her to expect you to come up with something good for her hair and appearance each time. It doesn't have to be something that will cost her money each time either. That can definitely work against you if she starts thinking that each time she sees you she's going to have to fish for her credit card.

When you have her back in the shampoo bowl next Thursday, use a different conditioner on her and tell her you are. Say, "Janice, I'm using conditioner X on you today. Usually, I use conditioner B on you, which works really well, but I have another client with hair similar to yours and we used X on her and it really made a difference. I want to see if it will do the same for you."

Always, every single time you see every single client, look at them with this thought in mind: "If I could do anything and everything I wanted to this client to make her look absolutely the best I am capable of making her look, what would I do?" Then, propose those things, or at least one or two of them. So many times, we take our clients and the services they request for granted and never suggest that highlight to them that would make them a knockout.

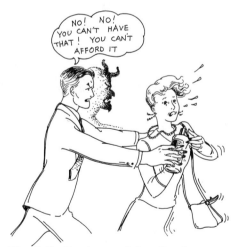

Fig. 4.6 Don't spend the client's money for her.

In the very first consultation, keep that thought uppermost in your mind. I'll even tell the client, "I'm going to look at you as if you were my wife or girlfriend, and come up with the look I think would be the absolute best for you, regardless of what it takes." I will many times suggest not only a change in cut and style, but a perm, color effects, hair care products, skin care, and several other services or products. It is up to the client to say no—*don't spend her money for her.* We say this over and over, and still cannot say it often enough. *Don't spend the client's money for her.* Suggest *everything* that will serve to give her the best look she can have. She may not buy the entire package (although she certainly *may*), but she will buy part of it now, at least, and chances are good to excellent that she will end up eventually getting everything you suggest. For starters, you have planted a seed in her mind that will grow and grow until she will be asking you, weeks or months down the line, "Do you still think highlights would look good on me?"

After a client has made five or six visits, then it's time to suggest a more substantial change. Change is the fashion businesses' business! Do you think Liz Claiborne keeps trotting out the same dress every spring? Sometimes, however, it becomes difficult to come up with new ideas by yourself.

In our salon, most of us have worked together for some time and know many of each other's clients, at least by their faces. At our weekly sales meeting, one of the sections is devoted to changing our clients periodically. Each stylist prepares a list of clients who are due in that week to whom they would like to suggest a change, and asks the others for suggestions on what might look good on that client. We get lots of great ideas from one another, and the process is yet another component in the synergy we seek to create within our staff.

It also gets each of us in the habit of really looking at our clients and seeing new possibilities. And it kind of puts each stylist on the spot to come up with their own list of clients to suggest change to, creating what we consider to be a good habit.

We don't expect to see each client changed either. Many won't, but that's all right. Just the fact that a change was suggested by her stylist imprints on her consciousness that her stylist is the person to come to when she *is* finally ready for something different. Our salon doesn't necessarily put out looks radically different from other salons in town, but we do have the reputation for being on the cutting edge, and this was no accident. We wanted that reputation and took the steps necessary to obtain it. It wasn't happenstance and almost never is.

From time to time, quiz your client as to her satisfaction. Are you doing all she desires with her hair? Ask her *fun* questions, such as "If you were on a different planet, how would you like to wear your hair?'' Or, ''If you were single (if she's married) and dating, how would you wear your hair? Would you change it?'' You'll be surprised at the responses you get, and it will give you a lead into suggesting changes for her.

Just remember, so long as that client comes to you, you owe it to her to be consulting with her. Think of yourself as her doctor. Anticipate her needs before she does. Practice preventive hair care. Look for symptoms of dissatisfaction. When she tells you, ''I wish my hair were a little fuller,'' don't laugh and say, ''Don't we all!'' and go into a discussion of what you did on your date last night. Get excited and tell her how she can have exactly what she wants. Design ways to get out of her what it is she's really thinking. Show her five pictures of five different hairstyles and ask her which ones she likes the best. When she picks out a couple of them, look for things in the hairstyle she might not have noticed that made those models look especially lovely. For instance, she might have picked out three photos that all have subtle highlights. Point this out to her and tell her what similar highlights will do for her. This is just one example of what can be countless ways to create positive change in your clients—and put more change into your pocket!

When you have clients that have expressed a desire to achieve a particular goal with their hair, say, growing out the length until it's at the shoulder, don't assume your job is over at that point, and that from now on all you'll need to do is maintain it at that length. Once a goal is reached, let the client enjoy it for a month or two or a bit longer, and then begin suggesting a major change, perhaps even going back to shorter hair. Change is the backbone of the fashion business, and staying too long with the same look or style renders that person out of style. Girls with great legs, who were ecstatic when miniskirts were the rage, may have been disappointed when longer hemlines came in, but believe me, they adjusted the lengths of their skirts to fit the new lengths. Hair is not any different in most ways from clothing styles, and the client should be educated to this philosophy. Get them in the habit and mode of thinking that lets them expect and enjoy change.

And when a client is ready to leave the salon, whether it's after her very first visit or her ninetieth, plant a seed in her mind that will set up the next sale.

''You know,'' you tell her, as her hand's on the door, ''I can see a few subtle auburn highlights in your hair when the sun hits it that I didn't see under the fluorescent lights. Why don't you think about adding a few more to your hair when you come in next time. Just think about it, and if you decide you want to try it, plan on an extra forty-five minutes.'' Then, say your goodbyes and walk away. You've planted a seed and it will grow. When she gets into her car, she'll look at her hair in the car mirror and try to visualize those highlights, and she'll think about it many times during the next few weeks. In effect, she'll sell herself on the idea you've planted in her mind.

Don't leave it at that though. Go immediately to her file card and make a simple notation, "Suggested auburn highlights." Then, when she comes in, ask her if she's thought any more about your suggestion. You'll be amazed at the percentage of those who will ask for whatever it is you've suggested. Many times, if you've suggested a highlighting or a perm in such a manner, they're back on the phone to you the next day asking if they would have to wait until their next scheduled cut to receive the highlight you suggested, or can they get it sooner!

Try it, it works!

And remember, consulting with the client never ends until she no longer is a client.

REVIEW

1. *Proper physical layout of the consultation area:* Make a professional impression. Make the area clean, neat, uncluttered—no macramé, kiddy photos, fuzzy bunnies—and think about utilizing some of the new advances in video and computer simulators.

2. *The psychology behind a successful consultation: Your* client wants someone in authority to tell her what she should do with her hair. She secretly wants to be in the audience of the Phil Donahue Show and have a renowned stylist make her over. She knows she'll be putty in the right person's hands. Make her realize *you're* that person (you are!). Establish yourself as the professional.

3. *Understanding what the client is after:* She wants to be as attractive to herself and others as possible. That's it. Simple.

4. *Timing the consultation:* Be in charge and follow a set program. Visualize what you want to accomplish and how you're going to achieve that—what it will take. Time is money. Overlong consultations are counterproductive. Ten to twenty minutes should be maximum.

5. *Direct the consultation:* Be in control and provide the lead. Set yourself up as the authority by the way you come on and the body language you use, make your diagnosis, give it and explain why, and ask for the sale. Even though you are under a self-imposed time limit, don't let the client see this. Keep the conversation flowing, but in the right direction at all times, eliciting the answers you want by the way you present them, and never let the client feel hurried or pressured. Easy!

6. *Understand that consultations don't end when the haircut begins:* Consulting with the client continues throughout the entire lifetime of the client–stylist relationship, until it finally ends, if it does.

CHAPTER 5

How to Use Magazine Photos and Other Visual Aids

CHAPTER LEARNING OBJECTIVES

The stylist successfully mastering this chapter will know:

1. *When to use photos and when not to.*
2. *Avoiding the situation of picking a style.*
3. *Computer simulations: pros and cons.*
4. *Using photos to educate the client.*
5. *The power of the proper photo and the limitations.*
6. *How to use a photo to sell your styling idea.*

As the ancient Chinese proverb (or was it Arabian?) says, "A picture is worth a thousand words." That is a partially true adage; to make it more correct it should perhaps read, "The right picture at the right time is worth a thousand words."

We are most certainly a visual society, and this is assuredly a visual age we are in. Most of today's population has grown up with TV and even the older generations were exposed to movies early on. Some even predict the book, as we have always known it, will be obsolete or at least relatively rare within the next few decades, a prospect I shudder at. At any rate, pictures, whether animated as in television or movies, or in print, have proved to be an extremely valuable medium, and as such, are a very useful tool within the modern hairstyling salon.

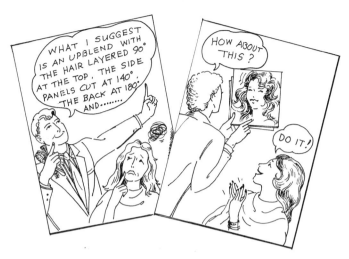

Fig. 5.1 One picture or one thousand words?

There was a time when I was young and full of myself, when, if a client brought in a picture of a style she desired, I became offended. I was a *creater*; I didn't do *other stylist's styles,* I did *my* styles. Pictures were an insult. Ah, but we live and we learn! Mark Twain commented on a stage most of us seem to have to go through, when he said something to the effect that, "When I was eighteen, I thought my father was the most ignorant man alive; when I turned twenty-one, I was astonished to see how much he'd learned!"

Pictures of styles have their place in every salon. That is a statement few might find fault with. The trick is to know when to use them and when not to.

One time *not* to use them is when the consultation has gone exceedingly well, and you and the client are both on the same TV channel. When you *know* you both have the same mental image in mind, and you know her hair will do (with your help) what she wants it to do, don't cloud up the situation by introducing another element; i.e., by introducing a photo of the style at this time. You've *made the sale;* don't lose it by overselling, and that is what whipping out a picture at this point risks doing.

Usually, the proper time to introduce photos into a consultation is when your verbal skills have failed and not before. At this point, the right photo can speed matters up and get both of you pointed in the right direction.

When you do bring photos into the consultation, an important rule is to not introduce too many choices. Two, at the most three, different looks are plenty; more than this confuses the client, especially if she begins to like five, six, or even more of the pictures. It's like turning a starving man loose at a smorgasbord and telling him to have whatever he wants. The more he sees, the more he wants, and the more he wants the more undecided he becomes, and eventually

59

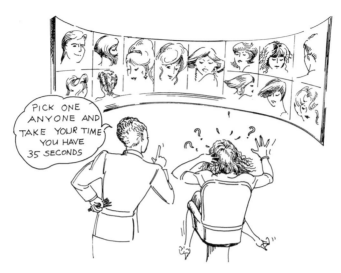

Fig. 5.2 Too many choices can lead to nervous breakdowns.

he runs the risk of a nervous breakdown before he ever takes the first bite. Give him the choice between a hamburger and a cheese omelet and he'll pick one or the other and be happy.

Presenting too many photos of different styles creates a situation wherein the client has too many variables to integrate in making a good decision and she ends up *picking a style,* which most times results in the wrong decision. Frustrated by too many choices, she ends up by questioning her choice, a frame of mind not conducive to a happy result. An old German adage says, "Too many ducks muddy the pond," and thus it is in this instance. Keep it simple, stylist (KISS), and you will have a pleased client.

An innovation, in recent years, that has great promise, is the introduction of computer simulations. Software programs are available that allow you to show the client what various hairstyles, hair colors, etc., will look like on her, and they can be terrific selling aids. There is a downside, however. Most of the programs I've viewed seem not to have been designed by a hair designer; the styles shown seem to be stilted and unimaginative and mostly dated looks. As the science becomes more progressive, it is expected the quality will improve, so keep an eye out for new developments. Another problem is giving the client false and misleading expectations. Showing a client who possesses one of those fine-haired heads (ten thin strands per inch) a photo of herself with thick, luxurious tresses, can only lead to a confrontation in which you will have to inform her of the reality of the situation. *She ain't never gonna be able to have that style!* As long as you remain within the bounds of reality, considering her hair texture and other drawbacks and only exhibit styles that you can procure with *her* hair, you should be all right.

For hair color changes, computers can be great. We all know how difficult it is to exhibit what a different color will look like to a client once it is applied. Holding that tiny sample swatch to her present hair as she sits before the mirror has led to many a tense situation when she views the final result, even though the color is exactly as you showed her. That color, that seemed so great to her in a two-inch swatch placed against her head, looks totally different when applied to her entire hair. A facsimile on the monitor before you start gives her a much better idea of what will ensue, and can help both you and her to make the right decision.

Be careful here, too! If you think you might not come up with exactly the same color exhibited on the screen, prepare her for that. Based on your experience with your color line and the results you usually obtain on particular client's hair, don't mislead her into thinking she will get hair exactly the color the monitor exhibits, if you think there might be a difference. Explain that individual hair colors may react differently, and although you will be getting very close to the color shown, it may not be exactly that color.

Being a colorist is fun and exciting, but there is a problem many of us have when tinting clients, and that is sometimes we end up with more warmth in the final result than we had anticipated.

Thia Masciana of the International Color Exchange reminds us "The best way to avoid problems in hair coloring is to test-strand your formula before you apply it to your client's entire head."

She gives a handy mixing method for such strand tests: "Substitute small measuring spoons for your mixing bottle or bowl. Create a miniversion of your formula using the exact proportions you will use in your final formula. There are three teaspoons in a tablespoon. Usually you can make a test formula with a total of two tablespoons of product. Process it the full time required by the manufacturer so you have an accurate result. The full color development will *not* be apparent in half the processing time. No one can accurately predict a color result without pretesting. One half-hour of pretesting can save you hours of redoing and a lot of grief. Your clients will appreciate your precision hair coloring, just as they appreciate your precision design work.

"The hair color manufacturers offer guidelines for creating color formulas. However, these are only *guidelines*. Only pretesting will show you accurately whether or not the formula you've created will achieve the desired result."

Now, I know all the color experts claim that if you simply follow their directions the color will *always* be exact, but that is simply not always the case. Sometimes, we happen upon clients with odd problems with their hair, and the color does not perform as we expect it to.

Recently, I started tinting a client's hair. She informed me she had never had a coloring she liked, but she kept getting it tinted because she hated her gray. Even though the color effects she had received hadn't been satisfactory, they were better than the gray. Being the expert colorist I imagined myself to be, I supposed that she had just been the victim of colorists who were unfortunate enough to not possess my vast coloring experience.

I got surprised. Ungrammatical, perhaps, but that's what happened—I got surprised! The ash color I applied came up quite warm—*red,* in fact! After stripping it, and going through several hours of strand tests on her hair, I discovered that warm shades turned ashen in her hair. This broke all the rules as I understood them, and I was completely puzzled until I began playing detective with her. After a lengthy, probing discussion, I discovered that she was a heavy *night sweater,* and that she was going through her change of life. The reason her hair had been reacting adversely to color, I reasoned was related to the hormonal activity on her hair and the change in the electrolytes in her system related to her excessive perspiring. Whatever the underlying cause or causes, we came up with the right color. The fact of the matter is, that no matter how good a colorist you are, there are at times, special circumstances that will skew your anticipated results. Performing test strands is the way you can foresee major problems such as the one I encountered and minor ones can be forestalled with a little preparation.

The most common complaint I have seen over the years with clients in color is that "There's too much red!" Clients are terrified of red. Actually, it's normally not red they're afraid of, but brassiness or an unnatural tinge of orange, because we all know there's no such thing as red in hair color, only various shades of orange. I have yet to come across a stylist who hasn't fought with several clients over the *red* in her freshly tinted hair.

There is a simple solution that will almost alleviate the problem completely. Take a few minutes prior to applying the color and explain the strand test to the client and explain how permanent hair color works on natural pigment. When natural pigment is acted on by peroxide and ammonia (the two active ingredients in permanent hair color), it lightens and turns slightly warmer. The depth of the natural pigment is the clue as to how much warmth you will encounter. In other words, the darker the natural hair color, the more red, orange, and gold you will see as you lighten. This advice comes from Thia Masciana again, who also reminds colorists, that, "It is wise to point out that most brown hair reflects warm highlights. If a true ash or drab color is desired, the natural pigment must be prelighted. Using a lightener, lift the natural pigment to one level lighter than the brown color desired. Shampoo that product out of the hair. Then, apply the ash brown tint. With this method, you are eliminating enough of the naturally occurring warmth. You will achieve a true ash or drab brown.''

Ms. Masciana also states that many clients will choose not to invest the time or money required to eliminate all the warmth from their hair. Explaining what is involved in this procedure, she says, gives a client a more realistic expectation. Giving your client accurate information eliminates surprises!

I show the client two color swatches, both the same color and level, one ash and one warm, and let them pick the one they find the most flattering, first telling them that both are the same color. It is an eye-opener for most of them, and almost every person will select the warmer color as being preferable.

Try changing your client's expectations to a more realistic one and you'll end up with a pleased and loyal color client.

Another problem with color is that the color she was so excited about in a one-or two-inch swatch looks very different to her when completed. There are several reasons for this. One is that we all get used to seeing ourselves in a certain way, and when we drastically change, we see the result tenfold more than what it really is. If you have a client who wants her medium-brown hair back after twenty-two years of gray hair, that medium-brown is going to look like coal-black hair to her. Be certain that the color she is asking for is really what she wants.

When a client's hair turns gray, that follicle has lost the ability to produce pigmented hair. That loss of pigment is not exclusive to the hair. When our hair grays, our skin becomes lighter, and our eye color becomes lighter also. We lose pigment throughout our whole body. For this reason, the color we had as adolescents or in our twenties is no longer appropriate.

Another reason for disappointment with color is that even though the color matches the swatch or example shown, once it is all over the head it imparts a different value. How many have had the experience of finishing a coloring, proud as a teenager who's licked acne, and had the client wail, ''That's not the color you were going to use!'' Then, when you put the swatch up to her and showed her it was right on the money, she still wailed, ''Well, it doesn't look the same all over!'' *I've* certainly been there!

We get smart too late sometimes, but after this has happened a few times, it's time to readjust our thinking, and figure out how to avoid this problem in the future. A good way to do this is do just a little less than what the client indicates she wants, unless you're totally convinced that she knows exactly what she wants. When that new color client, who's never had her hair tinted, asks for that pale, pale blonde, take her hair just a little darker. When that middle-aged grandmother wants to return to the medium brown of her teens, take her to a light brown first, or at least a bit lighter brown than what she thinks she wants. This is where the art of coloring comes into play. The science is relatively easy; the art takes a bit of time and experience!

Keep all this in mind when using computers or other aids, and don't expect them to be a *miracle in a box,* but what they are, a very effective visual aid, when used with a bit of common sense, applying experience where needed.

As the people who design computer programs become more astute about the art of hairstyling and more attuned to the fashion aspect, these programs will only get better and better. Be aware though, that styles change yearly, and that great program you paid thousands of dollars for a year ago, may be virtually useless and out-of-date very quickly. Investigate what the company will make available to update the system each year and what flexibility is built into the program, as you can end up with a very expensive piece of equipment that sits idle in the back room.

Educating our clients can be aided greatly by the judicious use of photos. As we seek to make the language more precise between client and stylist, thereby increasing the quality and ease of communication, pictures can be an invaluable aid. For instance, describing the angles and cut you propose to employ in creating the style, you may want to show her photos that illustrate what the result will look like.

A good example is *layering.* Many times per week, a client will seat herself before me and desire a new style, and I have determined that the ninety-degree layered cut she walked in with needs to be changed to a different angle. I will explain as best I can how I will achieve this, sometimes holding a large comb up to illustrate the angle to be cut, but clients aren't hairdressers and this method is unclear at times. When the average client hears the word *layered,* she has a preconceived notion of what that is, and the concept most clients have of *layering* is the old *shag* angle. She doesn't realize that this is only one of hundreds of degrees possible in cutting and that virtually all styles are layered, albeit at different and various angles. This becomes a common source of confusion and can tie up precious time while you try to explain what the style will look like. The proper photo at this time will save time and explanations.

Even though the client may not fully understand the theory of angles in haircutting, I feel it important to explain them to her. If nothing else, she will realize that I am not just picking up hair and chopping it off, without rhyme or reason; that there is a method to my madness, and that she is in the hands of a competent stylist who is thinking through the project. This is but one more way to establish yourself as the authority and the person in charge, especially because many stylists don't do this. In the client's mind, the stylist who approaches her with the view that he or she is going to educate her as to why he or she does things a certain way, is the consummate professional and the stylist she has always wanted to go to.

There used to be a philosophy and saying in the hair business, that, "You can't (or shouldn't) sell your hands." Old-timers in the business will remember it well. What it meant was, that you shouldn't educate the client too much or she would learn enough that she didn't need you any more. We kept all of our *secrets* from her. The philosophy stems from the days in which most clients were getting roller sets and combouts and had to come in weekly to get their hair *arranged.* Only the stylist knew the combination, and the client was a virtual prisoner to her hair. The car windows had to be up at all times, even in the sweltering heat of August (even in cars without air-conditioning), and swimming in the lake was out of the question. She could go in up to her neck, but that was it. Shower caps were worn, and some went so far as to buy satin pillow slips so as not to muss their hair. Stylists during this era were genuinely concerned that their clients not figure out how to do their own hair, thereby eliminating the need for a professional, and that is where the attitude developed.

Unfortunately, the attitude still pervades in some circles, and it is counter-productive to the client's needs today. There is little chance that if you educate a client about what you are doing to her hair that she will go home and try to duplicate it herself. If she does, you can be assured that she will be in forthwith, to have you *fix* it! And, similarly there is a small chance that she will take the knowledge you have passed on to her, go out and open a hair salon down the street, and become your competition. Ridiculous as this sounds, that still seems to be the attitude of some stylists today.

Believe me, the stylist who takes the time to explain what he or she is doing and why, will, in short order, become one of the busiest stylists in the area, and not necessarily *be* the best stylist—just the best *professional.*

The right picture at the right time, is indeed, worth a thousand words. The wrong picture at the wrong time can, on the other hand, lead to a disaster. Beware of the pitfalls of picture situations, such as presenting too many choices, presenting obviously impossible choices, or presenting style choices totally inappropriate to the client and her face shape and/or lifestyle.

Use photos properly, that is, to illustrate what the style you suggest will look like on her and to help make the final sale. When the client is *on the cusp,* the right picture will take her over the edge and into the direction you wish her to take. Pictures, used judiciously, can be one of the most powerful selling and styling tools within the salon. Used improperly, they can lead to nervous exhaustion, tension headaches, and premature baldness, not only in the stylist, but in the client!

REVIEW

1. *When to use photos and when not to:* When the situation calls for it and not otherwise. When you *know* both you and the client are tuned to the same TV channel in your minds, don't cloud things up by introducing new elements. When she is unclear about what you are trying to get across, a picture can be very valuable, but keep in mind that two, or at the most, three choices are optimal, and more than three choices can cause a nervous breakdown.

2. *Avoid the situation of picking a style:* Don't offer a smorgasbord of styles; the client will become surfeited and an intelligent, reasonable choice becomes impossible. Also, any decision reached will be constantly second-guessed by the client, and she will be constantly wishing she had picked the contents behind *door number sixteen,* instead of the ones she choose behind *door number twelve.*

3. *Computer simulations—yes or no:* Yes, if the program used is up-to-date, fashionable, and fits the limitations of the client's hair. No, if these criteria are not met. When purchasing a system, check into what the suppliers of the program do to keep the product updated.

4. *Using photos for client education:* Powerful illustrations for showing what you want to do in the style and to illustrate differences of cutting and styling techniques. Also, a good way to show the client how the same cut can be styled in more than one way.

5. *The power of the proper photo . . . and the limitations:* Use the right photo to reinforce your idea to the client and give her a concrete mental picture of what it is you want to do for her. Don't use photos that will confuse the issue and create obstacles to a mutually acceptable goal.

6. *Using photos to sell your styling ideas:* When that client is *almost* convinced of your suggestion, the right picture will seal the deal.

CHAPTER 6

How to Convince Your Client to Change Her Style

CHAPTER LEARNING OBJECTIVES

The stylist successfully mastering this chapter will know:

1. *How to create the impression in your client's mind that you are the person to come to for change.*
2. *How to make your client want to change.*
3. *What is change? Is a change always drastic?*
4. *Some of the common obstacles encountered in changing your client's hairstyle and how to overcome them.*

As ours is a fashion business, and as the keystone to fashion is change, it is imperative that we understand this and use it to our advantage. We can take a page from the clothing industry, which is closely related, and use their techniques to make ourselves successful.

I have never understood why a woman (or man) who wouldn't dream of wearing the same dress style she wore three years ago to the annual company bash would not hesitate at all to comb her hair into the same style she wore *ten* years ago. It doesn't make any sense!

Yet, it happens all too frequently. The fault lies with many of us in the hairstyling profession. We don't encourage the client to change.

But you can bet the clothing industry does! Oh, and do they! Not only *every year,* but . . . *every single season.* And why? Because they recognize that

67

change creates need. That's why hemlines go up and down; why shoulder pads are in one season and all of a sudden they're passé; why blue was the predominant color, the *only* color last year; and why now if you're not into brown and muted shades, couturiers snicker at you.

How many people keep their clothing until it is worn threadbare and no longer useable? Not many, in your acquaintance, I'm sure. We don't change clothing because it is no longer serviceable, or warm, or we don't like it any longer. We change because it's out of style. Pure and simple, we march to arbitrary whim, even though the arbitrary whim is created by someone we don't even know.

Purists, or at least people who consider themselves purists may rebel against this, but they don't seem to make many inroads against the changing fashion scene, at least in the clothing portion of it, and although someone who insists on "being his or her own person" as far as clothing styles may be someone to admire for their independence, they had better not try to make their living designing blouses. They may have integrity (in their minds) but almost certainly will have little or no income.

The same is true in hair fashion. Sadly, there are those of us in this business who resist change and fight it valiantly. Without knowing so, they are fighting the very fabric and heart of their industry and dooming themselves to a low income and slim client base. For change in hair fashion is what keeps the client coming in the door, and when clients seek out new stylists, many times it is only because they seek a change in their hair and don't feel their current stylist can give it to them, or, worse, is not *willing* to give it to them. If you get nothing else from this book, studying this chapter alone and profiting from it will perhaps be one of the best things you can ever do for yourself, business-wise.

Change is inevitable. Recognize that and benefit; refuse to acknowledge it and suffer.

At one time, I owned a salon and employed a stylist as an assistant. I had misgivings at the time of hiring because of her appearance, but I hired her anyway because of her warm personality and years in the business. I should have heeded my instincts about her, based on her appearance, because it would have saved the unfortunate consequence of having to discharge her eventually.

What was wrong with her appearance? It was her hair. It was this long, long stuff, totally without shape or style, and it hung below her waist. Now, I have nothing against long hair and even prefer it on those who wear it attractively, with a shape and style, but in her case, such was not true. It was just . . . long hair.

And her hair reflected her attitude. Very quickly, I observed her poking fun at photos in hairstyling magazines that weren't clearly at least ten or fifteen years dated. *Anything* that looked *avant garde* or at least current, she sneered at—and openly—to clients. What she was doing in the hair fashion business, I still don't know. It is true enough that all of us have opinions about style and fashion, but can you imagine a prominent clothing designer criticizing another designer's style because it wasn't dated enough? It would be the kiss of death to her reputation as a fashion expert.

The same is true in the hair business. From time to time, I overhear hair-dressers laughing at something they have seen in a hairstyle book that looks different from something they are used to seeing. These are generally nice enough people, but they don't belong in the hair fashion industry. At least not with that attitude.

The long-haired hairdresser who openly made fun of *avant garde* styles was eventually asked to leave. I'm sure she felt I was a horrible person, even though I tried to make the parting a diplomatic and tactful one. However, there was no way she could remain in a salon that was dedicated to fashion when she was so against it. She had come from a situation where she had been earning less than minimum wage, even though her talent was prodigious, and she returned to a similar situation, and, although I don't know this for sure, blamed her situation on everything but her attitude toward hairstyles. There were just enough clients out there that shared her attitude and patronized her so that she had a little bit of business, but that's all it will ever be as long as she adheres to the concept she has of fashion.

If you are of the same persuasion, it might benefit you to take a long, hard look at your attitude and see if it might not be holding you back.

Let us assume it to be a *given* then, that change is important to our industry and to our own personal success. How do we convince the client in our chair that it is in her best interest to update her hairstyle occasionally, especially when we know from experience that many of our clients are recalcitrant about such changes?

If it is a new client, the chore is much easier. Sometime during the initial consultation or during the performance of the service, you might do as I do. I say to her:

"You know, I firmly believe a person should change their hairstyle periodically. It is to a woman's best interest to change her look at least every six months. That doesn't necessarily mean a *drastic* change, but even a minor change achieves the purpose.

"Look at it this way. Let's say you have this green couch in your living room, and every week, fifty-two times a year, you move the couch and thoroughly sweep and clean under it. But . . . you always put it back in the exact, same spot. Do you know what happens? The couch becomes nearly invisible!

"Your appearance does the same. After you've worn the same look too long, those around you begin not to notice you any longer. I don't really think you want your husband to take your appearance for granted, do you?

"There is the other extreme, also . . . when you change capriciously every time something new comes along. That can show you have no style or mind of your own and is just as bad as *never* changing! Change doesn't have to be major nor does it have to be extreme to be effective. If you part your hair on the left, for instance, changing it an inch higher is a change and will be noticed.

"Because I realize that to change is difficult for many of us, and because I honestly believe it important to do so, I do something to kind of jog you into such changes.

"On the file card you filled out when you came in, I will keep an exact record of what we do to your hair. Except for one thing. I never write down how I air-form your hair. The reason I don't, is that I don't want to remember exactly how I dried it. From time to time, when you come in, I'll recommend a change for you and tell you why I think you should do what I suggest. If you agree, fine, but if you don't, each time I do your hair, you'll get a slight change, by accident, just because I won't know exactly how I dried your hair four weeks ago. If I can't get you to make a change, I can always duplicate your cut exactly, because I *do* record how I did that, but I won't remember how I dried your hair. That way, for one day you'll get a slightly different look and if you like it, great. If you don't like it as well, then nothing's lost because I cut it the same, and you can go home and duplicate it yourself. I think that's a nonthreatening way to get in the habit of changing periodically, don't you?

"I tell this to each of my clients, and so far none has disagreed with my idea. Is it all right with you?"

I then await her answer, and of the thousands of clients whose hair I have serviced and asked this, *not one single client has ever asked me not to;* not one has ever insisted I record how I air-formed and dressed their hair!

People *want* to change; they just don't want a disaster. They will readily accept minor changes; it is major, drastic, mind-bending changes they are most afraid of, and perhaps rightly so.

If you approach your clients in this way, you will have established yourself in their eyes as *the* person to come to for a hair-styling change. They won't leave you for someone down the street when they finally get so tired of the same old look they've worn that they're on the verge of upchucking. They'll see you as just the one to give them a different style.

Many of our problems in our business (with our clients) can be solved with a bit of forethought. We *know* clients leave stylists when they desire a change. Each and every one of us has had a new person sit in the chair for the first time simply because she was ready for a change and her old stylist wasn't. By anticipating that each one of our current clients will reach that same point, plan right now to nip it in the bud with the means I've suggested.

It's the same with product sales. So many times, stylists have hung onto their old product lines when other, newer lines have passed them by, quality-wise, because they think, "Gosh, I've just got that client convinced Brand X is the best—how can I switch her to Brand XY?" The solution is simple. Always prepare your client for such a change. (There is more on this technique in Chapter 10.)

Whenever you encounter problems with clients, realize that you will always encounter such problems, unless you work right now to forestall and prevent them in the future. When you encounter the client who is dissatisfied for *any* reason, sit down that evening and figure out why she is dissatisfied and think through how you can avoid the complaint in the future. Actually, you are fortunate if she complains to you, rather than takes her complaint to a new stylist. By complaining to you, even though it may make you uncomfortable at the time, she is presenting you the opportunity to rectify the situation and, therefore, retain her trade.

By the same token, when new clients come to you and voice displeasure over something their old stylist has done, search yourself and your methods to ensure that you aren't perhaps doing the same types of activities to your existing clients. You probably won't make the same exact mistake the new client has related displeasure with, *with her;* make doubly sure you aren't making the same mistake with others!

Talk to your clients about change. Educate them as to the value of changing their hairstyle periodically. Point out to them, gently, that clothing styles change rapidly, from season to season and from year to year, and the clothing we wear isn't even the prime focal point we notice when we view others. The hairstyle is.

Remind them that the first thing we notice about another's appearance is their hair. Say, "Think about how we describe a stranger to another. Don't we usually say something about 'the girl with the shoulder-length blond hair.' Or, 'You know her; she has the spiked red hair with the double-base'?" We *describe* others by their hair and hairstyle more than any other way. This is proof of the importance of our hair and also of the importance of keeping it current.

Ask them to pick up a fashion magazine and pick out any famous model. Ask them to consider the fact that an Elle MacPhearson may be seen in countless magazines wearing dozens of different outfits, but she always looks attractive. Why? Her hair has a lot to do with it. Her hair, like that of other successful models, is crucial to that success, and part of the reason she is considered beautiful and attractive. Her skin and hair are as crucial as the clothing she is modeling, and your clients need to know that the same is true of them.

Besides, it's just plain fun to change hairstyles! Both for you and for the person receiving the change.

Back up your philosophy of change. Every so often, every five or six visits, step back and take a long look at your client and actually propose a change. Treat them as a brand-new client, even booking extra time for that session. They'll never feel that they're being taken for granted, once you begin to do this.

And, if you have been cutting an individual's hair for some time without changing it, don't worry about frightening her with a suggestion of something different. Odds are, she's been itching for a new look but didn't want to *inconvenience* you by asking for your ideas. Many times, we give off vibes to our clients that say, "Look, I'm busy. Don't bother me with requests that will take more time than I normally give you." Although we don't come out and say that verbally, we oftentimes deliver that message in other ways. Be sure you aren't cutting one client's hair and overtly worrying about your next client, if you're on time and so forth. Remember the waitress, used as an example, who served the most patrons in the restaurant but never made them feel harried or hurried, and emulate her example. Don't create the atmosphere of being rushed and especially, don't ever, ever give the message that the client before you is a *burden* in any way. She will quickly relieve you of that burden, by patronizing someone not so stressed out as you appear to her!

Watch that longtime client's eyes light up when you suggest a change in her hairstyle. Don't expect each and every client to jump up, clicking her heels and scream, "Yes, yes, change me, change me!" It probably won't happen. Many such clients will gladly change at that time; many won't, at least not right away. But most will eventually. When you say, "Barb, I just came across a picture of a style in a book I think would look just wonderful on you. Let me show it to you and see what you think." If she doesn't agree with your idea of a change right then, chances are excellent that she will in the near future. You've planted a seed in her mind, and seeds have a funny way of growing.

Use intelligence when suggesting changes to the client. Extremes of any philosophy are usually bad, and the stylist who continually browbeats her clients into major overhauls is asking to reduce her client list. Don't set up a condition wherein the client begins to think, "Gosh, every time I come in she wants to remake me. I'd like to just catch my breath a bit and learn to do my hair the way it is and maybe even enjoy it awhile longer. I'm tired of my coworkers at the office running a lottery on whether I'll walk in with purple or green hair this week!'' Be sensitive to each client's particular psyche, and don't overstep the parameters of her particular boundaries of taste.

Have that resistant client thumb through a copy of *Glamour* or *Elle* or some other fashion magazine, and pick out who they think are the five *sexiest* models and who they think are the five *least sexy* models. Don't use the word *beautiful* or *attractive,* because nearly *all* the models will fit those adjectives, but specifically choose the word *sexy*. Have them bring in the ones they pick. This is an interesting exercise and one I employ often. Nearly always, the ones picked as sexiest have more contemporary hairstyles, and that is the only difference. It doesn't seem to matter if the model is scantily-clad or not; the hair makes the difference. Point this out to the client; draw her attention to what makes one of the two choices, both obviously attractive, look sexier than the other.

Then, suggest what she can do herself to look sexier. And, if you think you can't use the term *sexy* when dealing with older clients or with minister's wives or some other such category, think again! I don't think I could find a client in our salon, regardless of age or point of view, that wouldn't want to look sexier! I don't think you will either.

Sometimes a woman will *want* to change but doesn't think others whose opinion is important to her will like the change. How many times have you been told, ''Well, I'd kind of like to cut my hair shorter, but my husband hates short hair. He wants me to be able to trip over it.''

In cases such as this, gently explain to her the psychology behind hairstyles. Believe me, there *is* a psychology, particularly where length is concerned.

How many men have you known that insisted their wives wear their hair long, and then when you observe them at the cocktail party, they're flirting with the short-haired women? I'll wager more than one.

Long hair traditionally represents conservatism. In popular music circles, which singers traditionally wear long hairstyles? Country and western singers. Don't misinterpret me—I enjoy that music as well as many others, but country and western fans didn't get the reputation of being conservative for no reason.

And some men do like to have their wives and daughters wear their hair long. Long hair, for some, is *safe*. Short hair is rebellious. Think about it. Many a father has groaned when his little girl gave up her waist-length tresses for a bob. It signaled to him, the end of her innocence. The emotions behind hair length are strong.

But, is it fair? Is it fair a wife wears a style she doesn't care for, for her husband's sake, when she herself wouldn't dream of asking him to cut off those long sideburns she detests? Perhaps twenty or so years ago, but, as the

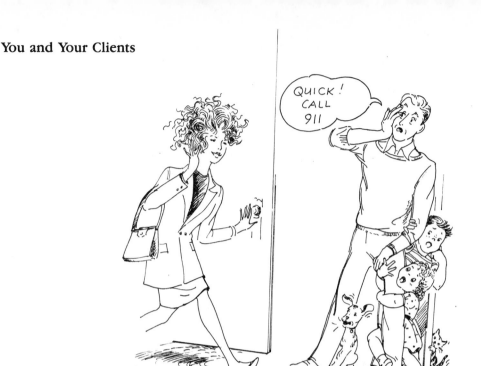

Fig. 6.1 Don't worry. Husbands, children, and small animals tend to settle down after the initial shock of a new hairstyle on Mom wears off.

ads say, "You've come a long way, baby!" Wearing a style you feel better about doesn't make you a bad wife or even a bad person. It merely makes you a *person*.

There's another fear behind a change in hairstyle, especially when it concerns a change in length. What is the first thing a woman does when a relationship goes sour? Doesn't she get a new hairdo and a new wardrobe? Haven't you seen that happen many, many times? Do you know why?

It's because there's a lot of pain associated with a relationship that's breaking apart. While you can't change the internal person and make the pain go away, you *can* change the outer person, perhaps in a secret hope that *that* will alleviate the stress, even though rationally you know it won't. But guess what? It really *does* make a person feel better.

Ever have an acquaintance who began cheating on her husband or boyfriend? What happens in those instances, oftentimes? Why, she gets a new hairdo and buys a new blouse and skirt in a color or style she never would have worn before.

When you begin to analyze it, it's no wonder husbands and boyfriends get anxious and feel threatened when the woman in their life begins to change her appearance. Subconsciously, at least, it signals that there could be something wrong with the relationship. Very young children get the same uneasy feeling when Mom cuts her hair differently. They sense, just as animals sense impending earthquakes, that something threatening may be afoot.

But guess what happens? After a week or so, husbands, boyfriends, and small children begin to settle down. It seems only Mom's hairstyle changed. Mom didn't. She's still Mom. And then everyone's all right again.

There is a certain psychology behind every hairstyle and hair length. The way hair is worn says something very powerful to everyone who views it. It categorizes us, stereotypes us, and classes us. It is important for those of us whose business is hair to recognize and understand the prejudices and biases of hair lengths and styles and to learn to educate our clients so they aren't unnecessarily ruled by those factors.

Everyone, every *normal* person that is, has a healthy desire to control those in his or her life. A small bit of this is healthy, but it becomes somewhat perverted when the urge to control becomes absolute. As long as a change of hairstyle remains within the bounds of propriety and fashion within the peer group and looks attractive on the person, who has the right to dictate appearance to another? There is a point to be made that we should want to look good to our *significant others,* and it is a point well taken and heeded within reasonable bounds, but many deny their own needs and desires when perhaps they shouldn't.

Point out some of these things to such a client, in as diplomatic a manner as you can, and perhaps she will become a candidate for that style you know would look terrific on her. At the very least, if you handled it properly, she may begin examining her relationships and begin making needed alterations in them.

If the client keeps throwing up obstacles and no matter what you propose you cannot overcome them, then accept the fact (to a degree) that she may never change, and be thankful for her business. But, don't take this totally for granted. From time to time, keep on suggesting new things to her. She may just surprise you someday by agreeing to what you propose. Continue planting seeds, with just a word, a brief suggestion, and many of the seeds you sow will grow, flourish, and flower eventually. Quite often, everyone in such a person's circle, has forever made certain assumptions about her, which may or may not be true. Sometimes all that is needed is a suggestion. She may have been secretly desiring a change, but needed the reinforcement of someone's opinion she respected to allow her to act upon her desire. Most of us, at times, are unsure about our own opinions and need such reinforcement for us to act.

Reexamine the change you are proposing to her. Perhaps it's a drastic change, at least in her view. If so, back off a bit and approach her with another suggestion, that's not so far afield. Ask her if you can try parting her hair a little bit differently, or if you can dress her hair slightly differently than you have been. When a person has worn a particular look for a long time, such changes that might seem minor to us will take on magnified proportions to her, but even so, won't appear too threatening.

Once you have effected *any* change on such a person, no matter how slight, it will be easier and easier to get her into something different. She will have discovered that the sky didn't fall and her husband didn't leave the Yellow Pages open to the listings for divorce lawyers. It will give her more courage to begin thinking about hairstyling changes.

Although there are some clients who will never change their hairstyle, it is to your advantage to be creating change in the vast majority of your clientele, because change is the very fabric and soul of our profession. When a salon

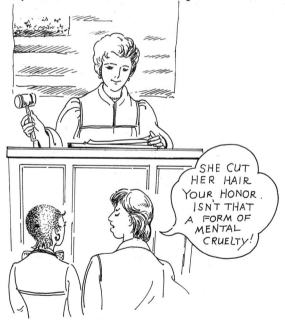

begins to change from being innovative and creative to being merely a *maintenance* salon, it is usually on the way down. Plus, how much *fun* do you think stylists have who keep on turning out the same dreary, outmoded looks day after day after day?

Preach change, practice change, effect change, not only in your clients but yourself. It's difficult to sell Cadillacs if you drive a Volkswagon. Show clients that you believe in what you're selling yourself.

When I get a particularly *tough nut* who resists change of any kind, what I will sometimes suggest to her is that she make an appointment with me for some day when she won't see anyone that day to just let me blow-dry her hair in a different way. I'll even do it for free. Such a suggestion takes the fear out of the experiment, because I'm not changing the cut, just temporarily giving her a different look. Some of the clients who have agreed to let me do so have become the fiercest proponents of cuttingedge fashion in the salon!

There is a catchall phrase that could very well describe the importance of changing hairstyles: "When you're green, you're growing; when you're ripe, you're rotten!"

REVIEW

1. *How to create the impression with your client that you are the person to come to for a hairstyling change:* First, be sure that you really believe that change is necessary for the health of our industry. You can't *sell* what you don't believe in. Then, begin immediately by sharing your belief with your client, that you feel it imperative that she change her appearance, even if subtly, every six months or so.

2. *How to make your client want to change:* By showing her the advantages. It will make her look and feel sexier and more attractive. It will keep her from appearing dated.

3. *What is change and does it have to be drastic?* Change can be so slight as an inch higher parting or a few highlights sprinkled subtly throughout the hair. With most clients, it *shouldn't* be drastic.

4. *Common obstacles encountered in effecting change:* Attitudes of others in your client's circle will influence her decision. If you feel her decision is not in her best interest, gently show her why you feel so, taking care not to get personal and perhaps even using a mythical someone else for your example or by talking in generalities, saying "men in general" rather than using her husband Sam as an example. When she begins to understand the why of those opinions, she may decide to change her own mind.

CHAPTER 7

Avoiding the Pitfalls of Overselling

CHAPTER LEARNING OBJECTIVES

The stylist successfully mastering this chapter will know:

1. *When zealousness is harmful.*
2. *Why overselling is detrimental.*
3. *What to do about it.*

Selling is the cornerstone of the hairstyling business. If a hair design is not first sold, then it can never be performed. Selling doesn't only pertain to the marketing of hair care products, it extends to every facet of the profession. A sale is made each and every time a client allows a hair designer to cut her hair and is remade each and every time she books her next appointment, for whatever service she desires.

There exists a certain antipathy against *selling* with a small percentage of our hairstyling fraternity. They seem to have the idea that *selling* a hair product or their services, is somewhat *beneath* them; that such activity is undignified, not becoming a *professional* such as they. Everyone is entitled to their opinion, but such an attitude can only lead to failure, for nothing, and I mean *nothing,* is moved within a hair salon unless it is first sold. In fact, the hairdresser who feels this way may not realize it, but he or she *sold* themselves to the owner or manager just to obtain a job.

Selling, whether it be a hairstyle, a house, or a used car, is a wholly honorable endeavor, worthy of the name *honest labor* as much as any other type of activity, provided certain ethics are upheld.

It is difficult to imagine any occupation that pays its practitioner a wage, fee, or salary that doesn't employ sales techniques to initiate the process. Without sales, we would operate in a vacuum. It would matter little how creative we are if first we did not convince someone to sit down in our chairs to show them. I suspect it is not *selling* itself that certain individuals resent, it is *unscrupulous* selling.

It is sort of like the story told of the famous politician's wife, who, while traveling in a plane and seated next to a reporter, was posed by him the rhetorical question, "Mrs. X, would you go to bed with me for a million dollars?" Upon a few moments reflection, she replied, "Well, to be perfectly frank, for a million dollars, why, yes, I think I would." To which he shot back, "Well then, what sort of sex would you give me for ten dollars?"

At that, she became indignant and haughtily said, "Just what kind of person do you think I am!" He looked at her calmly, and said, "Well, now, Mrs. X; we've just established what kind of person you are—we're just haggling over the price."

To some of us, the crime doesn't seem perhaps to be selling—it's the *degree* of selling.

Which leads us to one of the extreme degrees sometimes found in selling that can be not only somewhat unethical, but also disastrous to our goal of creating happy, delighted clients, and that is the crime of *overselling.*

Assuming that if you've read this chapter thus far, you're not a misguided purist that believes selling to be the next sin listed under the seven sins, let us then assume that you desire to be the best salesperson you are capable of. If that is so, beware of the fault of overselling. Beware, beware, beware!

More than any other part of the selling process, overselling is the most detrimental thing you can do, except maybe not even attempting to sell in the first place.

Ask any other selling professional what he or she considers the worst sin that can be committed when attempting to sell someone else a product or service, and the astute answer will always be, "Overselling!"

What is overselling? It's simple. It's continuing to sell something once the sale has been made. That's all it is.

What's the cure? Once the sale is made—shut up.

If nothing else is learned from this book, repeat this one phrase over and over until it is burned into your memory and you wake at night sweating, screaming these words. *Once the sale is made—shut up!*

How does overselling hurt you? Example: Mary, your client of ten years who has needed a perm for all ten of those years has just been sold—guess what!—a *perm,* by *you,* and you're in seventh heaven. You are about to effect a change upon her visage that you know will glorify her radiance and cause large numbers of attractive men to swoon at her now lovely countenance. You pick up the first rod, place the wraps around the combed section of hair, and . . . blow it. How? You make a statement. You make the *wrong* statement. You say, "Mary, I'm so glad you decided to get this perm. It's going to change your life. And, a great thing about my perms—this can last you up to six months."

As of this point, you're in deep water. You have just oversold the service. There may be remnants of permanent wave left in her hair at the end of six months, but it's not going to be the permanent wave result she will be anticipating. A major problem has just been created. Her trust in you is going to be completely shaken and perhaps forever removed, once she finds out her perm doesn't last six months.

I know you said the perm *could* last her up to six months, but she doesn't know you said that. What she heard you say was that it *would* last that long, and believe this or not, the way she will see it *lasting* is in pretty much the same condition as the first week of its life. Four weeks later, when it needs trimming to remove the weight and rejuvenate the curl, the first tiny doubts will begin to surface. It will begin to dawn on her that this perm isn't going to be around like you "told" her it would even two more months down the line.

It's tempting to oversell, especially when we want to make the sale so badly. We have just gone through a process where we've had to overcome twenty-six objections and when the client finally says, "Okay, go ahead," that inertia, or centrifugal force, or something, compels us to go on selling. We want to regard the difficult client with even more than we can give her. It's then that we lose something we've just gained—the *sale*—or we set ourselves up for a disappointed client sometime in the future, thereby negating effectiveness in future sales.

Overselling is a symptom of insecurity. Insecurity in our ability or insufficient faith in the product. When you attempt to persuade another to purchase something you yourself don't think worth the price, you will almost always oversell the product or service. If you find yourself overselling very often (we *all* do it occasionally), sit down and analyze what it is you're doing and why. Perhaps you feel uneasy about charging the price you do. If that is the case, try to determine if it is just your own insecurity about your ability (usually unjustified). Sit down with your manager or owner and tell them your feelings. Many times, a product or service that you feel guilty about charging what you do for it, turns out to be more than fairly priced, and someone with more experience can show you why it is priced the way it is.

If you are asked to perform services with products you consider inferior or substandard, have a meeting with your manager and tell him or her your concerns. Please keep such a confrontation civilized, and don't go in screaming that the perm you have to use is garbage and if only you had Perm XYZ instead, you wouldn't feel guilty about charging what you are. State your beliefs in a diplomatic way and ask if you might use a product you have more faith in. Allow too, for the possibility that what you have been asked to use may be of a higher quality than you are aware. If the manager or owner can explain this to your satisfaction, won't you feel better about having approached them? If this turns out to be the case, then you should feel a lot better about the price charged the client.

Look inside yourself first to be certain that this isn't just an excuse or alibi, and that what you are really having difficulty with is your faith in your own ability. This, too, can be overcome. Talking over those fears with the manager or a stylist you respect and trust will be extremely helpful. In general, it is not the quality of the product or service you are trying to sell that turns out to be the problem. Usually, it stems from the salesperson's lack of experience, which leads directly to insecurity. That is normal and that is common, but that is also totally unrealistic. Even if you have only a brief period of time under your belt as a hair designer, you already know volumes more about hair, the services

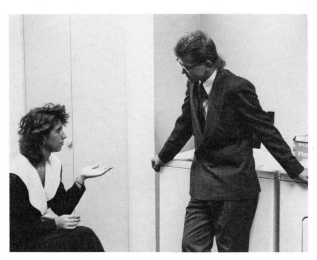

Fig. 7.1 Problem with a product or salon situation?
Talk it over with your manager or the owner.

performed on it, and the best products to be used in its care, than virtually every layperson. Although it is natural to feel uneasy about something that is somewhat new to you, don't let it keep you from doing your best and from charging a fair price for your labor and skill.

In addition, overselling can lead to heightened insecurity. Once a few clients like Mary come back screeching that their perms didn't last six months, or that their bottle of shampoo didn't last ten years, then instead of learning not to oversell, many times we end up overselling even more, just to mollify the client who's bent on embarrassing us.

In you anxiety to make the sale, keep in mind that what you are offering is of benefit to the client. You are not offering snake oil or miracle elixir. What you hold out to her is used by millions of satisfied people all over the world. You *know* what the product or service is and what it can do. Tell her that and nothing more. Don't make her extreme promises, even if you know of instances in which your claim may be true. If it is not the average experience, don't relate it. If anything, undersell a bit. Not so much that you lose the sale, but enough so that when the benefits manifest themselves to the client as being even more than what you represented them to be, you will have gained a client

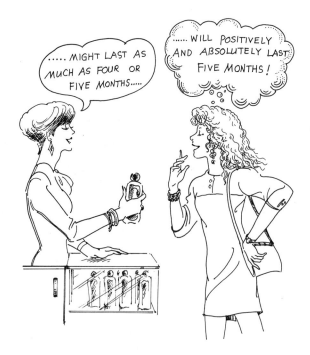

Fig. 7.2 People may only hear with half an ear and only hear what they *want* to.

that will trust you explicity from then on. When clients learn that you have represented something fairly and that it does all that you have claimed (and even more), then they will not only purchase virtually any product or service you recommend, they will also actively seek out and tell their friends about you.

Just remember. People hear with half an ear, and when they hear phrases such as "... may last as long as five months ...", what they *really* hear is "... *will absolutely* last five months."!

The basics of selling are simple. Suggest what it is you are selling to the client, give its benefits to her, and then *ask for the sale.* If she buys, give her the product and collect her money, or, give her the service and collect her money. If she puts forth an objection, counter with some more benefits or amplify the ones already given, and *ask for the sale.* If she buys, shut up, collect the money, and go on to the next one. If she has another objection, explain other benefits, and so on. Stop countering objections when you run out of *bona fide* benefits. She's not going to make a purchase—at least, not today. If you make the mistake of overstating the case, of promising more than the product or service can deliver, you may make the initial sale but you have most likely lost all future sales as well as her goodwill. You can't always sell everybody, but you should sell most of your clients most of the time.

If you haven't been overzealous and oversold the client, and she still hasn't agreed to the service or product, then quit. There is one final thing you can do before you let go. As she's leaving, just say, "Bye, Mary. Thanks for coming in. I hope you like you hair. It looks really good on you. And say, do me a favor,

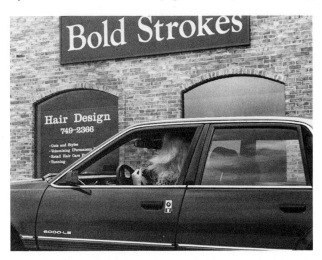

Fig. 7.3 Plant a seed!

will you? Just think about what we talked about, about highlighting your hair. Just think about it and mention it to your husband and see what he says. Okay? Thanks, and have a great day."

Then go on to your next client. You will be pleasantly surprised how many times that client who was such a tough prospect will call back in a week or so and ask if she can have the service you sweated blood trying to sell her. Sometimes people just need space in which to consider your proposal. If you haven't oversold her, then you will have maintained your integrity and will feel good about performing the service or handing her the product. The power of suggestion is just that. It is a *power!* Plant the seed and watch it grow. You'll see such a client go out to her car and pull the rearview mirror over to her and peer into it, and you *know* she's trying to imagine her hair with the highlights or perm you suggested.

Tell the truth, ask for the sale, and *don't oversell!*

REVIEW

1. *When zealousness is harmful:* When the client is given misleading information about the product or service, and expects more than can be delivered. You are setting up an unhappy client and probably a confrontation.
2. *Why overselling is detrimental:* It destroys customer confidence in you and your products and services and creates an unfavorable reputation for you as a professional. The reputation it creates for you is unsavory and counterproductive. It gives clients the distinct impression that you are unsure of yourself and what you are promoting.
3. *What to do about it:* Tell the truth, give the benefits without sugarcoating or inflating them, ask for the sale, and then—*shut up!*

CHAPTER 8

How to Convince the Client to Send You Her Friends

CHAPTER LEARNING OBJECTIVES

The stylist successfully mastering this chapter will know:

1. *The single most important element in building business.*
2. *The importance of persistence.*
3. *How to custom-tailor your clientele the way you want it.*

There are literally dozens, if not hundreds, of ways in which to build a clientele base in the hairstyling business. The single most effective way is to have your present clientele help you. What you will learn here may seem almost too simple to be true, and that is right. It *is* simple—as simple as most great ideas are—and, as foolproof and effective.

Many new stylists believe advertising to be the key to getting new clients into the salon, especially new clients for *them*. The new member of the staff asks, "Why don't you advertise more? If your advertised more, I'd be jammed up." What they fail to realize is that although advertising can be effective (although many times it is not worth the effort, if done improperly), there is a way to build their clientele right under their very nose, which costs nothing but a little effort and is a hundred times more effective in obtaining new clients than almost any other means.

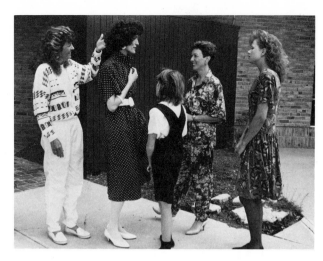

Fig. 8.1 Ask your client to send you her friends.

That is simply asking for the client's help. It goes like this: When the client you have just finished is ready to leave, thank her for her business and hand her three cards and say, "I'm glad you like your style and thanks for trusting your hair to me. I'm going to give you a few cards and ask you to send me your friends. Would you do that for me?"

That's it. That's all you need to do. Simple, eh? You'd think so, but know what happens? The new stylist will listen to you explain this and nod sagely that she understands completely, and the next time you see her at the desk saying goodbye to her client, she is saying, "Bye now, and here's a couple of cards."

It doesn't work that way! You can't just stick a couple of cards in your client's paw and expect her to do anything but file them in the circular file. They just won't send you a friend, unless you make a point of *asking* them to.

"Help me out. Send me a friend." It takes your saying that for them to do it.

Half the time, they don't know why you're giving them a card, unless it's to be sure they don't forget the salon phone number. When three cards appear in their mitt, they may assume you believe them to be the type that loses things and that giving her three means that even if she loses one or more she'll still have another.

Clients are not stupid, no matter how I've made them sound, but they do need direction. How much direction? One hundred percent direction! When a new client enters our salon, the receptionist or salon coordinator knows she is expected to point physically to the seat the client may take in the waiting room. People really don't know what to do unless you tell them.

When I see a stylist hand the client her business cards without saying anything, I remember an incident that happened in one of the first shops I ever worked in. It was a former barber shop that had decided to go *unisex* (remember that term!). *Unisex* always makes me think of a white horse with a cone growing out of the center of its head and possessing both sex organs.

Anyway, the owner of this shop had a sales ploy we were required to use called a *hogshead*. I never did know where he got that term, and it wasn't one of my all-time favorites, but you know how it is when you work for someone else . . . you do it their way.

What a *hogshead* was, was a white card similar to the cards you bought in high school for the cafeteria, that got punched each time you used it. This particular little dandy had ten punches on it and you put the client's name on the top and each time he or she received a service it was punched. When the last punch was made, she was eligible for a free service, and balloons would go up, jazzy music would blare forth, and a guy in a striped blazer and a straw hat would come out and congratulate them. That's not entirely true. The part about the free service was but the rest I made up.

I hated it. I hated *hogsheads*. I had nightmares about them. From an early age on, from birth, I think, I have detested the idea of giving something away, especially my labor. I have this weird idea that one is entitled to a fair wage for their work, and the idea of *hogsheads* went entirely against all my principles. But, I wasn't in charge of this particular circus, the owner was, and I, but a lowly employee, was required to participate in the "*Hogshead* Sales Program."

Well, I did . . . when the owner was present. When he was absent, I kind of forgot to hand them out or punch them unless the customer asked me to. There was another downside to these things. The client could use them with any stylist they wanted to, and there were days when all I did were *hogshead* clients that normally went to other stylists. All in all, it wasn't a good experience for me.

I had voiced my opinion of the things as twenty-year-olds are apt to do, but to no avail. The owner stubbornly resisted my very convincing arguments that we deep-six the idea of *hogsheads,* and I just as stubbornly refused to give them out unless he was present.

One day, when I had just completed my fourth *free* hairstyle in a row, all on customers who had never sat in my chair before, my fifth client of the day was seated before me. The owner was there that day, working right alongside me, and when I finished doing the client's hair, I knew I was going to have to present him with one of those little white monstrosities.

I had had it. I decided then and there that this was going to be the last *hogshead* that ever passed from my hand to another's.

When the client got up, I handed him a *hogshead* and said, "Here's your *hogshead.*" That's all I said. He looked at it in his hand and said "What's this?"

I said, "It's a *hogshead.*"

He said, "Oh."

Then, he said, "What do I do with it?"

I said, "You bring it in each time you get a style and we punch it."

He said, "Oh. *Then* what?"

I said, "We punch all the holes out. All ten."

He said, "*Then* what?"

I said, "Then, we give you a new *hogshead.*"

He said, "Oh," paid his bill and left.

That is an actual, honest-to-goodness account of what happened, with no embellishments whatsoever. Of course, the owner had a talk with me in the back room shortly afterward. And, of course, I made a job change, relocating in a salon in another part of town, but I often wonder about that client. Did he ever come back and get his card punched and what happened then.

The point is, the client oftentimes doesn't have a clue as to what she's supposed to do with the business cards you hand her, *unless you tell her.*

If you do this properly, she will send you her friends. People want to help others; they just need to be asked.

I have done this wherever I've gone as a hairstylist, in every single salon, and it has never failed to generate a bustling clientele. At the present moment, I can't think of a single one of my present clientele that hasn't sent me at least one friend, and there are several of my clients that have sent me twenty or more. It works.

There is another element to consider when asking clients to send you their friends. Be persistent about it. Many times a stylist will start out doing just what we ask her to, hand cards to the client and ask for her help, *but after a* few days or weeks quit doing it. You can't *quit handing* out cards and expect your business to grow. You *must* be persistent and do it every single time, without fail. Or, the stylist's business begins to fill in and she gets satisfied and quits asking clients for their help. If you're booked two months ahead, you still need to do it. It will ensure that you'll stay booked two or three months ahead and allow you to raise your prices. It's the best way to get a raise.

What you're doing is what every successful salesperson does. You're soliciting referrals. Ask any prosperous insurance salesman what his or her secret is, and invariably they'll tell you, "referrals." When they are making a hundred thousand a year, do you think they say, "Well, that's enough, I'll just concentrate on what I've got."? No sir. They know they have to continue getting referrals to maintain a hundred thousand dollar a year income and get even more if they want to make two hundred thousand. If you're opposed to making more income and buildng a bigger clientele, then don't hand out business cards and ask your clients to help you out. They won't. Not nearly as much, anyway.

Once you've built a solid clientele, then you can begin to shape it the way you want it, by the way you hand out cards. People generally tend to associate with others like themselves, both in personality and in temperament. Recognizing that, concentrate most of your efforts on those clients whom you enjoy and don't put as much effort into those you don't.

For instance, I personally prefer doing women's hair over men's. The reason is that I find women's hairstyles to be infinitely more varied and complex, whereas most men's styles tend to be more conservative and similar. One of the reasons I enjoy hairstyling is the diversity, and women's styles give me that much more than men's. Therefore, I very rarely ask a male client to send me his friends, whereas I always ask women.

My wife Mary, on the other hand, enjoys the ease of men's styling, and consequently, makes more of an effort to get them to send her their friends. As a result, she does about thirty percent male clientele whereas mine stays at about ten percent, percentages we both feel comfortable with. And the men I work on tend to be more experimental in their approach to their styles, whereas Mary's male clientele is composed more of businessmen. Neither is *better* than the other, just what each of us prefers, and we have each arranged our clientele in that fashion by deciding whom to hand cards out to and whom not to.

Indeed, in our salon, as in many, you can determine the personality of each individual stylist without ever meeting them, by merely observing six or seven of their clients. Each stylist has carved out their own cadre of clients by using this method. Knowing you've got a client list you enjoy to come to work to makes life infinitely more enjoyable!

I don't hand out cards to each client every single time she comes in, either. This can get old to the client. But I do occasionally, about every fourth or fifth visit. Another good time to ask the client to help you by sending you her friends is when you've made a major change in her appearance, when you've done a service you haven't done before on her, such as the first time you highlight her hair, perm it, or change her cut. Always be sure she has cards at those times, as her acquaintances will always comment on the change, and it provides an excellent opportunity for her to recommend you.

Take a page from that successful life insurance salesperson you know. When you are effecting that major change on that regular client, ask her, "What friend of yours could benefit from highlights such as we're giving you now?"

She'll think of at least one immediately. This is a golden sales opportunity. Seize it. When she mentions a name, don't let the opportunity slip by. Tell her, "Listen, would you do both her and me a favor? Show her your hair and tell her you thought of her when you saw the results—that highlights are something you thought would look attractive on her too, and you told your stylist about her and he suggested you send her in for a consultation." Make up a card with the friend's name on it, and write on it, "Free Consultation," and have your client give it to her. When a day or two has gone by, and you think enough time has elapsed for your client to have passed on the card, phone the friend and personally invite her to the salon for a consultation.

Salespeople of all kinds agree that the hardest part of their job is *prospecting,* that is, garnering new names to approach to sell their services or products. It is also the best source of new clients. Don't let a single opportunity to gather new names pass you by. Ask each client who can help you to do just that— help you!

Make it a goal to get at least one name for each client in the next week. Ask for the name of a friend of theirs who they think would enjoy and benefit from your services. Get their phone number and address, if possible.

You can even prepare a mailer to send to those referrals, which might say something like, "Dear Eloise Brown: Kathy Smith, a valued client of mine mentioned you the other day when we were discussing her hair and she felt you might enjoy visiting our salon. I would like to make your acquaintance and tell you about some of the services we provide. Please phone me at 555-5555,

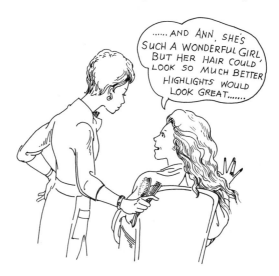

Fig. 8.2

your convenience and schedule a free consultation. After speaking with Kathy, I think I have a great idea for your hair. Thank you.''

Whenever the client sitting in your chair mentions that friend or acquaintance at work, that ''needs'' you, be sure and give her a card and ask her to present it to that friend. And, if she mentions more than one such friend, don't be shy. Get every name she gives you. The well won't run dry, believe me!

For those clients who make a practice of sending you friends, do something nice for them. Perhaps you might present her with a free bottle of shampoo on one of her visits, or give her a free blow-drying session, or even a cut and styling occasionally.

When I worked at Kenneth's in New Orleans, he had a special promotion that increased business significantly. He had a special business card printed up that was presented to each client. A notation was made on the card each time that client sent in a friend that hadn't visited the salon before, and for each five friends sent in, the client received a free style. Some clients sent in so many of their friends that they went months and, in some cases, years without paying for their services!

He also ran a salon competition for the stylist with the most referrals. Various prizes were awarded weekly, ranging from dinner for two at some of New Orleans' world-class restaurants to TV sets and VCRs. It was a huge success. Two methods of determining winners were used. The stylist with the highest *percentage* of referred clients won one contest, and the stylist with the highest *number* of new referrals won the other, on a weekly basis. Sometimes the two aren't mutually inclusive, and a newer stylist with fewer bookings could compete fairly as well as the busier, more established stylist.

Referrals are the lifeblood of the business. Elsewhere in this book are outlined various other ways of generating new business and clients, but the person seated in your chair is the single most important source of new clients.

Half the sales job is done if she is pleased with your work. When you ask your clients to help you out by sending you their friends, what you have done, in effect, has been to create a sales staff. Each and every one of the clients you ask to refer their friends is a sales person for you. If you have one hundred clients, you should have one hundred sales people in your sales force. It lessens the work you will have to do for one thing, and it doesn't take higher math to figure out the potential of one hundred salespeople, each selling your product (you) to a friend. It's a much higher success ratio than what you by yourself could generate!

Make it easy for your clients to make referrals. Take only basic information such as name, address, and phone number. If it requires much effort on her part to come up with more than the name, don't have her do it, unless you are

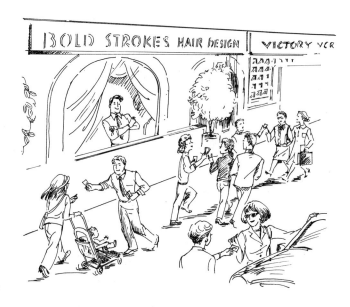

Fig. 8.3 Each of your clients should be part of your personal sales force.

fairly certain she won't find it troublesome. Get the name and look up the phone number later yourself. Then, follow up. Call or send a mailer right away.

Assure the client that you will treat her friend as well as you treat her. Let her know that if she refers a friend to you, her friend will have cause to thank her for the fine job you are going to do for her.

At a salon I owned years ago, I had the following message printed on the back: "The highest compliment you can pay us is for you to send us your very best friend." The message got across, loud and clear, and many people commented on it . . . and most sent us their best friend!

I've even told people, "I really enjoy working on your hair and I enjoy your company. I've noticed that people tend to attract as friends others who are much like themselves. It would be wonderful to have a clientele such as yourself. If you have any friends like yourself, please send them to me." It works. Hardly anyone is immune to flattery, especially heart-felt and honest flattery, and clients will respond to comments such as this. Doesn't it make you feel good when someone tells you they like you? It works the same for your client.

Just remember: People *want* to help out others, especially if they like the person, and even more specifically, *if their help has been requested*. Try it, and keep on trying it.

REVIEW

1. *The single most important element in building business:* Ask your clientele to help you out. Hand the client three cards before they leave and physically *ask them to help you out—send you a friend.* The number of cards given is important. Two cards is too few, and more than three (unless you sense the person won't resent it, or unless she asks for more) is presumptuous. You want to give your client the impression she is *helping you out;* not single-handedly building your business for you. Of course, if she requests more cards, don't be stingy!

2. *Persistence is important:* Don't hand out cards for awhile and then cease doing so. Even when your book is full, keep on handing out cards. Persistence will pay off, to the point where the book will become so full you'll have to raise prices in self-defense! A great position to be in.

3. *Customizing your clientele:* When asking clients to help you out, concentrate on those clients you like doing the best. Like attracts like, and chances are good that the client's friends are much like her. If there is a certain segment of the population you'd like to build, concentrate on those clients that represent that segment, more than you do others. Don't necessarily neglect other types of clients, but give your strongest sales approaches to the segment you wish to build the most. Be careful here though. The client you can't stand, but who loves your work, may send you a friend of hers that is so unlike her, you would have never had the opportunity to meet her and retain her as a client if you hadn't asked for the referral.

CHAPTER 9

Where the Money Is: Extra Services

How to Sell Perms, Color, and Other Services

CHAPTER LEARNING OBJECTIVES

The stylist successfully mastering this chapter will know:

1. *The "numbers" that demonstrate the value of extra service income.*
2. *Which clients are prime candidates for extra services.*
3. *Selling techniques.*
4. *The philosophy of "not spending the client's money for her"—why it is so important to always remember.*

There are two ways to go about creating a career in hair designing. There is the *smart* way and there is the *not-so-smart* method. Of course, we know which path *you* will take. . . .

In almost any endeavor of human activity, the main precept is to perform "less work for more money." There is nothing inherently wrong or immoral about this precept; it is merely the more intelligent way to conduct life's business. This is the basic concept behind most labor unions and nearly any other work-related organization or fraternity. We, as humans, have finite boundaries—

boundaries of time, to be precise. We are limited by so many working hours in a day, a week, a month, a year . . . and a lifetime. Which is better, to work eighty hours a week for four hundred dollars pay, or to work forty hours a week for a thousand dollars? The answer seems obvious!

Because of the finite limitations of time God or Nature has placed upon us, it is to our advantage to work less for more rewards. One of the ways to achieve this in our profession is to create a need for extra services, such as permanent waves, color and highlights, nail care, skin care and makeup, tanning, and so on. As these are ordinarily higher-ticket services, the more permanents we give and the more highlights we perform, the higher our gross dollar income will be; that is, provided we have priced these services properly. A service that takes more time and more education and skills should be charged for at a higher rate, and the additional cost of supplies or materials should also be factored into the price.

For instance, if your charge twenty five dollars for a normal cut and style, and it takes you a half-hour to perform this service, and it takes you two hours to perform a permanent, a hundred dollars is not the right price to charge. After you take the cost of the permanent itself into consideration, plus the additional knowledge required to update perming techniques, you would lose money by giving a perm at that price. You would make better use of your time by giving four haircuts and styles. So, price your extra services so that they

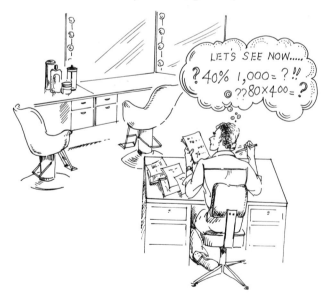

Fig. 9.1 "Now, which is better, eighty hours a week for four hundred dollars or . . . ?"

reflect these factors. If you perform other services simultaneously, for instance, cut a client's hair while a perm is processing, you can take that into consideration, but remember the public is accustomed to paying a higher fee for a more specialized service. An office call that takes fifteen minutes in a doctor's office may be billed at twenty-five dollars, but if a gall bladder is removed in a surgical procedure and the procedure takes thirty-five minutes to perform, your bill is not going to be based at the rate of a hundred dollars per hour! Take a page from other professionals. The client is not only usually expecting to pay more for extra services, but is also willing to do so, in most cases.

Let's take some numbers that illustrate the value of increasing extra services within the salon. For purposes of illustration, let us create arbitrary prices and time limits for each service. (These prices and time limits are *only* for purposes of illustration and should *not* be taken as recommendations for what *you* should charge. Depending on your level of ability, demographics, clientele, and other such factors, you may be higher or lower.)

Let's say that we are going to be charging twenty-five dollars for a cut and style and that it takes us a half-hour to provide that service. Let's then say that we are going to charge a hundred and twenty-five for a permanent wave, and that it takes two hours to give this service. Let us also assume we will be working forty hours in a week and that we are fully booked. The cost of the perm we will be using is five dollars. (There are other costs to be figured in, in both haircutting and giving a perm, but for sake of simplicity, let's just assume a flat five dollar cost for the perm.)

With this assumptions, let us further assume we have two stylists in our salon, Bob and Gail. Both are booked solid, using all available time, but the difference is, Bob does no perms; he's a *cutter* only, and he is able to give eighty cuts at twenty-five dollars each. He will gross two thousand dollars for his work week. Gail, on the other hand, talks up perms with her clients, and, as a result, does ten perms during the work week and forty haircuts. Her gross will come to two thousand, two hundred and fifty dollars. Both stylists were equally busy, but Gail earned two hundred and fifty more dollars. If she had wanted to, she could have booked an additional cut with each style, while the perm was processing, and earned another two hundred and fifty dollars. Even figuring in the additional cost of the perm, which would have been fifty dollars, she picked up an extra two hundred for the week for the salon.

There are some other benefits Gail enjoyed that Bob didn't. She didn't have to have as many clients as he did (fifty clients, compared to Bob's eighty clients), so advertising and marketing costs were lower for her than for him, and the ten clients who received perms had different (and more) needs for retail items which she sold them (and received a commission). Plus, her work appeared better, enhanced by the perm, which should have resulted in those ten clients being a more positive advertisement for her services. And so on and so on.

This is all fairly elementary, but sometimes it helps to reinforce the apparent value by putting it down on paper and looking at it. Any time you can service a smaller number of clientele and make the same or more gross dollars, you are doing something right!

Now that we all agree as to the value of performing extra services, who are the candidates for these services?

Everyone that walks into the salon.

Everyone.

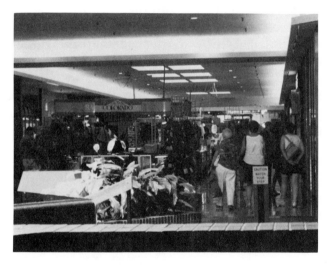

Fig. 9.2   Everyone that walks into your salon is a candidate for extra services.

There isn't a client entering your establishment that wouldn't look better with a perm, color, or highlights, a little tan, manicured nails, the right makeup, a slimmer body from a body wrap, or a more refreshed sense of being from a facial. Can you name anyone from your present clientele that couldn't benefit from one of these services or any of the other services we are qualified to perform? I seriously doubt it.

So how do we sell our perms and color and facials? By asking them to buy. And there are a number of ways to do that.

Suggest, suggest, suggest.

"Hi, Mrs. Jones, howareyouhowarethekidshowsyourhairbeendoinghaveyou-everthoughtwhatafewhighlightsinyourhairwouldlooklike?"

Suggest to the client services you feel would benefit her. Tell her why you've made the suggestion. *Show* her what her hair would look like with the service. Place a small color swatch in her hair and ask her to imagine how gorgeous she'll be with highlights. Show her a picture of the same style she's wearing but with a perm. Show her the eye color she needs, the fullness she'll receive from a wave that she doesn't get now. Talk in terms of *benefits* to her. "Auburn highlights will make your eyes sparkle." "A body wave will give you fifteen extra minutes in the morning you can use for *just yourself.* You won't have to use a curling iron any longer."

Ask her if she's ever considered any of your other services, and if she has, ask her if there's any reason you shouldn't book her for that service, or, time permitting, let you do it right then and there.

Sometimes price is a factor and the reason clients don't ask for certain services. They're fearful it will be more than they think they can afford and they're embarrassed to ask the price. At one time, there was a prejudice against posting service prices within the salon. It's time to rethink that philosophy. Many times, not having prices prominently displayed loses business for us. A great many times, the price of a permanent is lower than what the client assumes and they would have gladly gotten one long ago except that they just

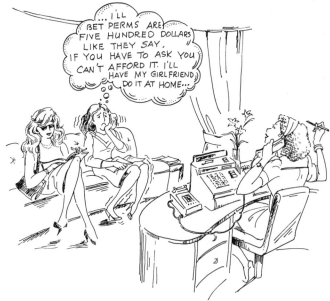

Fig. 9.3 Are you losing extra services business because clients assume the price to be more than it really is?

assumed it would be much more. And just having all your services listed, along with the fee, lets them know you *offer* these services. They may not even realize you do highlights, even though they see others in the salon giving them. People aren't as observant as we think, sometimes. Or, they may think everyone else does highlights in the salon, but *you* don't. Let people know what you offer and how much it is.

Develop easy, quick ways to introduce new services gently to reluctant clients. If your client balks at the idea of a major highlighting, suggest lightening three or four subtle pieces at the bang area at a lower price. Get them introduced to the service painlessly and create the habit for them of thinking about other services for their hair. Suggest a temporary color or even a shampoo color for the client who's not yet convinced she should try permanent color. Take that male client and use a curling iron on his hair to give him an idea of what a body wave could do for him.

Use synergy within the staff. Teach your stylists to compliment each other's clients on the looks you've given them and to suggest other services for them. When Nancy has just given her client, Beth, a perm, walk by and say, "That's a beautiful perm, Beth. Your hair looks great. A few highlights would really set it off, now, wouldn't it, Nancy?" We do things like that all the time in our salon and it generates even more business. Many times, the stylist has already mentioned the same thing and when another stylist comes over and suggests it too,

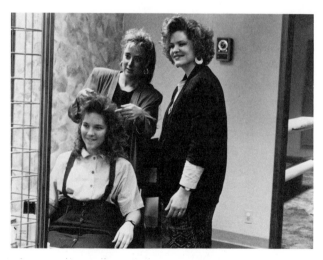

Fig. 9.4   Synergy works! Compliment your fellow stylist's work and *"accidentally"* mention another extra service that would make the client's hair look even better.

the suggestion is reinforced. People sometimes find it difficult to make decisions. They want and need reinforcement from others, not trusting their own ability to decide. When two people seem to agree on the same thing, quite often, this is all that's needed to tip the scale in favor of the sale. Major, successful corporations have known this for a long time. That's why they often hire prominent personalities to endorse their products. Upon analysis, what makes a famous basketball player's opinion on the "best tasting beer" more valuable than anyone else's similar opinion? Nothing, but the technique works. People need reinforcement in making buying decisions. Advertisements are run hourly on the tube quoting so-called *studies* that claim "ninety-eight percent of doctors polled recommend brand X aspirin over all others." I'm reasonably certain, you could locate doctors to endorse virtually any nonprescription drug on the market, (for the right fee), so the validity of such *endorsements* is virtually nonexistent. So why do companies use such tactics? Because they work!

When the stylist who works at the station next to yours walks by and suggests highlights to your client, it has the same effect on her as the endorsing doctor in the TV ads does. It lends authority to your own suggestion, and, in her mind, she now has *permission* to buy the service. After all, two *experts* (you and your fellow stylist) have *both* recommended it!

Don't think you should only sell one extra service to the client, either. Recommend everything you offer that you feel would benefit the client. During the initial consultation is a great time to sell many of your services. My own philosophy, and one that I come right out and tell the client, is that I look at that client as if she were my own wife, and what I will recommend is *every single thing she needs to give her the best possible look.* Don't look at the client and think, "Well, she needs a perm, cut, and color, but she won't get all of those, so I'll try and talk her into the perm." You're spending the client's money for them at that point, which is probably the single biggest business mistake made in salons today. Don't make those buying decisions for your clients. They are perfectly capable of saying no to something they can't afford—they really don't need your help in doing so. *Never* assume they can't afford something or won't want it. Assume they *can* afford the service and *do* want it. *Always.*

So much income is lost because of attitudes we carry. How many times have you seen a stylist sell a bottle of shampoo and then recommend the client "try a small bottle first"? Try a *huge* bottle first! If your product is so good, and you believe in it, then isn't *more* better? Why, sure it is. They save money! Isn't that the whole idea? Isn't that why that stylist probably recommended the smaller sized bottle? To "save" them money? Well, that misguided stylist isn't saving that client money, unless he or she assumes that's the last bottle of shampoo the client will ever need. Sooner or later, if the product is good and the client likes it, which I assume to be the case, then she will need another bottle. In the course of a year, she may need the equivalent of two gallons of shampoo. Which is a cheaper way to purchase two gallons of shampoo, in eight-ounce bottles or in liter bottles? You see, even that stylist who thinks in his mind he's saving money for his clients by recommending smaller bottles is, in reality, costing them money. It's to their advantage to buy larger amounts.

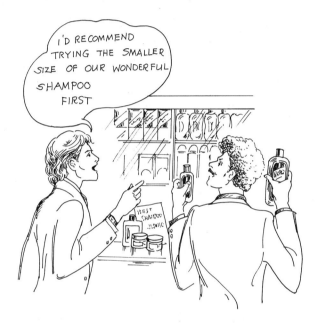

Fig. 9.5 What's wrong with this picture? The prize, should you guess correctly, is *more income.*

The same is true of extra services. The reason they came to you and your salon is to look better. If you only do half the job, the cut and the perm, when you know what they really need is the cut, perm, highlights, the skin toner, the shampoo and conditioner, and the makeup lesson, then to only suggest the cut and perm is to only do half your job.

Try to understand the average client. They don't know what they need. They want you to tell them what they need. How many times have you had a client who said, "Some day I'd like to go to that (major, famous) salon for a total makeover." Or, if you already work in that major, famous salon, haven't you heard a client or two say, "Some day, I'd like to go to that (*other,* major, famous) salon for a total makeover."? Chances are pretty good that you have.

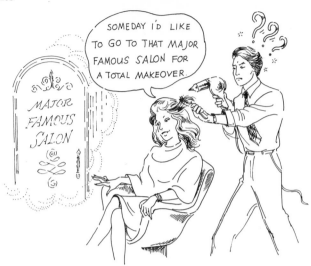

Fig 9.6

Listen to what they're really saying. What they're saying is that they're not happy with what you're doing to their hair. They want to look better. They want you to tell them what they have to do to look better, but you are perhaps too worried that they might say, "no." Big deal. So what if they say no? They may say yes. The odds are very good that they will. You've already accepted the "no" answer by not asking them in the first place. What have you got to lose?

If that client does go to that major, famous salon for that wished-for make-over, what do you suppose the stylist that gets that client in their chair will do? Do you think he or she will be thinking, "Well, let's see now. She has this two-year-old brown cloth coat so she can't afford highlights, so I'll just suggest a slight trim."? Ha! Don't count on it. One of the reasons that salon *is* a major, famous salon, is that they never learned to spend the client's money for them. They made the *client* say no. They didn't help them out by assuming they couldn't or wouldn't buy a service. They assumed that not only *could* they afford the service, they were probably frothing at the mouth to receive it!

Many times, when that client has said no, a month later she'll ask for the service. By making the suggestion, you've planted a seed in her mind. Like many seeds, it will flourish and grow. That's how we sell many extra services in our salon. Quite often, at the desk, after we've checked out the client and she's ready to leave, I'll say, "Thanks, Judy. Say, you know what would look good in your hair? Highlights! Think about it. Highlights would look great on you." And that's all I'll say. Many, many times, when she calls in for her next appointment, she'll ask if she can get highlights. If she doesn't, I'll reinforce the suggestion during the current service by bringing it up and asking if she's thought about it. If she has (and you can bet she has), then I'm into my sales pitch, trying to counter her objections, if any.

Stylists will sometimes say, "Well, I don't want them to feel like I'm trying to sell them something new every time they walk in the door (the client)." Well, surprise, surprise! That's what you're supposed to be doing—selling them something new every time they walk in the door! That's why we think of our salons as *businesses,* and not charitable enterprises. That's what businesses *do;* they *sell* things! Charities, on the other hand, *give* things away, but, unless you have inherited a great deal of money, and don't need any more, running your business from a *business* philosophy might be more advantageous than running it from a charitable point of view.

Look for openings and opportunities to sell extra services. That older client, who brought in the picture of Elizabeth Taylor and wanted the same cut, should have it pointed out to her that it's not just the haircut that makes Elizabeth Taylor look so great. It's also the hair color and the make-up. If she doesn't get all three, then how can she expect to even come close? It's in cases such as this that I will wish I also was licensed to sell contact lenses, because you can bet I'd be showing her the latest in the violet tints! When the client picks out a photo to show you the style she has in mind, point out the highlights in the model's hair or the perm that is supporting it and let her know that she has to have that also if she wants to approach the look desired. She also has to have the blow dryer or the heat rollers, the hair spray, the mousse,

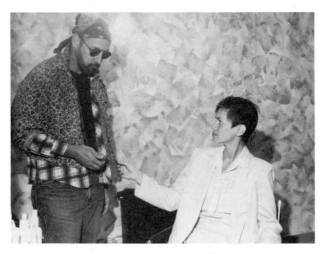

Fig. 9.7 Do you run your business like a business or a charity?

the glaze, and the once-a-week reconditioner! She also has to have the makeup application and the weekly facial and skin care treatment. She has to leave with some filled-up retail bags if she really wants that look and plans to maintain it.

Remember that client who often wished she could go to that major, famous salon and let that guy who's on the Phil Donahoe Show every four months do her hair? Well, she *went,* and guess what? She spent five times more there than she had in the last *year* in your salon, and although she may complain about it aloud, secretly, she's ready to do it all over again, next month. Chances are that she will, too. I've worked in all sorts of salons, from the tiniest salon in the tiniest village to some very well-known salons, and in the *name* salons I was fortunate enough to have been hired into, probably more than half of our business was very average people from smaller locales who felt they had to come into our salon to get what they had been hinting for or even begging for in their previous salon. Time after time, such a client would leave, after spending hundreds of dollars, and what I had done for her wasn't anything anyone else in any salon in the country couldn't have done and perhaps better. They just never suggested it to her because they were *spending her money for her.*

I worked at Michael and Company in South Bend, Indiana over twenty years ago when it was a strictly male salon. They were one of the best salons in town and charged the highest prices, and ninety percent of the clientele was Notre Dame students. Every single day, we each had student clients who literally counted out the cost of their style in change—in nickels and dimes and even pennies. They would save and save until they could afford a haircut at Michael's. All around us were budget salons, and they were busy too, but none was close to being as busy as we were. Anyone who works in a college town, on a student clientele, knows how *poor* students are. The point is, we didn't follow the philosophy of the rest of the salons in the area, who also catered to the students. We didn't try to spend the clients' money for them. We charged what we felt we were worth, listened to many of them complain about the price, and watched them painfully count out the money in silver . . . and then make their next appointment. Each time they came in, and they kept coming in and kept sending in their friends that were as student-poor as they were.

We sold them permanent waves and highlights and this was in the early and mid-1960s. Our perms in this period were in the range of forty dollars, which was high for the era and the locale we were in (I see salons today, in the 1990s charging less!), and we were catering to the clientele that had the least disposable income of any measurable group in town and Michael's kept ten stylists fully booked every day of the week.

If you offer quality work, people may gripe a bit about the charges, but they'll pay it. If they won't, there are others that will.

When I worked in The Crop Shop in New Orleans, the top stylist at the time, Janie, would gross several thousand dollars a week in services, and probably seventy percent of her gross would be in highlights. She was a marvel at highlighting, and clients I wouldn't dream of suggesting highlights to, were getting them from Janie. The chief reason she did so well and was the major star in the salon was that she wasn't afraid to suggest services for the client. For *every client*.

We forget sometimes just why it is a client comes to us. It's not just to *lower their ears*, but to enhance their appearance. When they upgrade the salon they are visiting, they are *excited* about their forthcoming visit. In their heads are visions of exiting the salon looking gorgeous, beautiful, *sexy*. How do you think it makes them feel when the stylist says, "Howdoyawantyerhair?" It's no wonder they balk at buying a bottle of shampoo, their expectations have already been destroyed.

We, sometimes, are looking at them in a different way. They are only number seven on our list of fifteen people whose hair we will service that day. They become *numbers* to us, and just another client to get through so that we can call it a day. We all get in this habit, but it's a disastrous habit to fall into. We need to remind ourselves about what the client expects and is looking for when she enters our doors. You are not "number seven on her list of stylists for that year"; you are the saviour who will finally make her look like the goddess she's always known she was. The time she spends with you is very important to her. She is going to see you only once every month to month and a half, and she expects you to treat her as such, not as "number seven out of fifteen." Hark back to that successful waitress who sees hundreds of people in a week, but makes each individual feel special and singled out for her charm and service.

Really think about and *get inside* the client's head. Imagine the thought processes that have brought her here, to sit in your chair, to await your magical ministrations. *Listen* to your clients. Haven't they said things like, "I told everyone at work I was coming here today. They're all waiting to see what I look like." Or, "Ruth (one of your clients) has told me so much about you. I hope you can do something with my hair." They're *excited*. And, perhaps you're looking at her and thinking, "I've only got forty-five minutes. What's the easiest and quickest thing I can do to her so I can get to my next one?" On *their* agenda are all the people they're going to run to and show their new look to, and on *the stylist's* agenda are the next clients. Is it any wonder many clients are dissatisfied with salons and stylists? I've even seen stylists treat that new client as if twenty were backed up and waiting, even though their next appointment wasn't for four hours! It just doesn't make sense.

We just become inured to what we are doing and forget what that client, new *or* old, is there for. We need to figuratively sit in the chair ourselves, once in a while.

Go to another salon and get your hair done and see how it feels to be treated as a number, to walk out with the same look as everyone else in the salon. Just don't tell them you're a stylist too, and you'll see what most clients go through in their sojourn in salons.

All of us get lazy from time to time. We fail to realize why clients are seated before us, and we need to remind ourselves of that. There may be a scene in your own past that can help you walk in the client's shoes when you need to. For myself, when I find myself taking clients for granted, I harken back to my high school days when hairstyling for men first came into vogue. There was a salon in town, the *first* salon in our town, that offered men's hairstyling, and much was said about this establishment. There were those who sneered at *men's hairstyling,* thought is *sissified,* and wouldn't be caught dead in such a place; and there was the other camp, who were interested in the ladies, who swore by the place. It took months for me to gather up my resolve and make an appointment, but finally I did. I couldn't get in for a week, and for a full

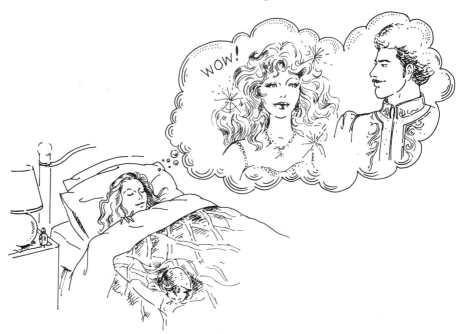

Fig. 9.8 Remember the anticipation and excitement you felt the first time you went to a really good salon?

week, all I thought of was my impending visit. I was going to look like a movie star or a rock idol! I was, by turns, excited, anxious, scared, and exhilarated! Finally, the big day came and I nervously entered the salon, expecting heaven knows what.

I wasn't disappointed. They shampooed my hair, which was a first; the barber always just whipped his clippers out and cut my hair in five minutes. The shampoo took longer than any of my previous haircuts! They even explained why they were shampooing (to break down the bonds of the hair for a more precise cut). They took me to another area (heavens! you went to more than one place!), where my stylist gave me suggestions as to how I should wear my hair. I didn't know what to say or how to answer him. He didn't say, "Wantyerhairlikelasttime?" I was in culture shock. Not being the connoisseur I am today, I let him have *carte blanche*. When he was done, having used an array of tools I was unaccustomed to seeing used on my hair, he placed a hairnet on me and placed me under an overhead dryer. When the hair was dry, there was not a hair our of place, which he made sure of by spraying it with hairspray. Hairspray on a man! This was 1958 and I was in absolute wonder and awe. When I left Riley's Hairstyling For Men (still open today and still one of the best and busiest salons in town and servicing more women than men), I was in Nirvana. I wouldn't even sleep in bed that night, but spent the morning hours sitting up in a chair so as not to muss up my style.

I must have gone through the four or five products I had purchased, reading the labels over and over, even though I was exhausted from running all over town and *casually* dropping in on certain gorgeous girls and other friends, and popping into establishments where I might be seen.

The next day, I nervously washed my hair and tried to style it the way the stylist had shown me. It worked!

My barber, good ol' boy that he was, lost a customer. Forever.

The point of all this is not simply to take you on a moonlight ramble down memory lane, but to illustrate to you how much a hairstyling session can mean to a client. Chances are, your first experience in a quality salon was similar. Draw upon that when you feel you are beginning to take your clients for granted and when they become "number seven out of fifteen." Clients, especially first visit clients, are hopeful and expectant of magic being created, and are in a frame of mind, if properly recognized, of going along with practically anything you suggest to them, if they are convinced it will make them look better.

Evert Riley, the owner and founder of the style salon I first visited, knew and understood this over thirty years ago, and still does today, which is why his salon has withstood recessions, style changes, and all the other forces that have caused other salons to come and go while his remains a leading salon today. Even today, when I walk into his salon, there is an air of excitement, and the young stylists working for him now emit a visible air about them that says, "Get excited—you're going to look wonderful when we're through!" And that is the atmosphere to create if we would be successful.

Remember the feeling you yourself had upon visiting the first salon that changed your appearance to that wonderful look, and suggest to your client whatever it will take to make them look their very best, no matter what it will cost them.

I've had clients laugh and say, "Man, you sold me everything but the kitchen sink!", to which I reply, "If the kitchen sink would make you look better, we'd be looking for a large enough retail bag to fit it into."

Sell extra services and always remember—*don't spend the client's money for them.*

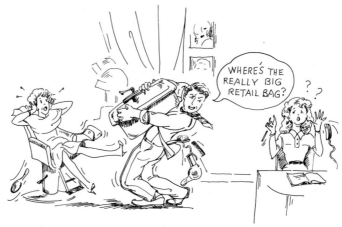

Fig. 9.9 Whatever will enhance the client's appearance, suggest it!

REVIEW

1. *The numbers that demonstrate the value of extra services income:* By promoting extra services, such as permanent waves, highlights, color, etc., you don't need as large a client base to achieve the same or higher gross dollars generated weekly. A stylist doing thirty haircuts per week and no extra services, will earn less than the stylist doing ten cuts a week and four perms and two highlights.

2. *Which clients are prime candidates for extra services:* Every client. Repeat: *Every client.* Say this over and over to yourself until you know the answer better than you know your own name.

3. *Selling techniques:* Suggest the service or services; ask for the sale; help out your fellow artists by suggesting extra services to their clients. Plant *seeds* in client's minds. Show the client the *benefit* of what you are suggesting to her. Watch for openings and opportunities, *windows,* to sell an extra service. If the client shows you a photo of a desired hairstyle, point out that the reason the hair looks so good in the picture is because of the highlights and perm the model has, as well as the cut and style.

4. *Don't spend the client's money for them:* Don't assume the client will say *no;* assume she will say *yes.*

CHAPTER 10

How to Convince Your Client to Use the Professional Products That Will Make Her Hair Healthier and More Attractive and Put $$$ in Your Pocket

CHAPTER LEARNING OBJECTIVES

The stylist successfully mastering this chapter will know:

1. *Why retailing is important not only to you but also to your client.*
2. *How proper retailing builds service revenues as well.*

3. *Effective selling methods that work.*
4. *Some alternatives to traditional retailing philosophies.*

Some of us have been in the hairstyling business long enough to recall when hair care products weren't even carried in the salon, and can remember a time when "selling" carried a bad connotation among many hairdressers. After all, we were *artists,* and not crass *salesmen!* It was beneath our dignity, or so we thought. Oh, we perhaps displayed a few combs and brushes and perhaps a can of hairspray or so, but, beyond that, not much else.

Those days are gone forever, and we should be forever grateful that they are. Thanks to some far-sighted individuals who began to show us the importance of healthy hair and how we can contribute to that health, more and more products began showing up in forward-thinking salons. We not only educated ourselves as professionals, but we also saw the wisdom of passing that education along to our clients, thereby making the health and appearance of their hair better, and also making our trade more of a profession, as now we not only cut, perm, and color hair; we *prescribe* the chemical concoctions that will enhance that hair.

Individuals such as Jheri Redding, Vidal Sassoon, Edmond Roffler, and many, many others, whose contributions have meant so much to all of us, showed us the value of understanding the physical makeup of skin and hair, and in doing so, handed us the key to unparalleled financial success as well as the key to gaining the respect of the public that patronizes the stylist.

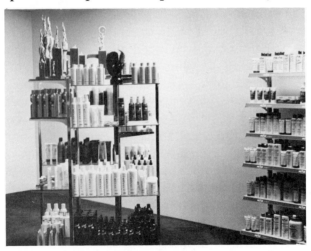

Fig. 10.1 The days when all we carried were a few combs, brushes, and a can of hairspray are gone forever.

When I began in the hairstyling business in 1966, the emphasis was on *hair-dressing*. Many hairstyles were horribly *hacked* and *chopped* and then *arranged*. By torturing, teasing, beating, and bending hair, we got it into contrived shapes and then loaded it up with clouds of lacquer to make it stay for at least a week, until the client came in again, to have it retortured into shape. We, as hairdressers, held the key to the style. There was no way the client could get her hair to do what we did. Consequently, women were slaves to their hair.

Literally, a woman didn't dare go swimming without protecting her hair from the water, or even have the window rolled down in a speeding car. Her *hairstyle* would be ruined, and she hadn't a clue how to get it back into the *style* her hairdresser had achieved last Friday or Saturday.

Hairdressers were slaves of a sort, also, in those days. Three-fourths or more of their business was transacted on Fridays and Saturdays, and the rest of the week, in the main, they just sat around the salon, doing each other's hair. When Friday and Saturday rolled around, they worked frantically, doing one client after another, for twelve- and fourteen-hour days, under incredible pressure. There would be a waiting room full of irritable patrons; stylists working in a frenzied haste on two, three, or even four people at a time; fans and air conditioners groaning under the load of smoking dryers as the beautician of the day scurried around yelling "Where's my next one?" as she tried to locate that client who had disappeared somewhere, perhaps into the restroom for a moment's respite; and other hairdressers working up an ulcer fretting about getting farther behind.

Not a pretty picture, but a fairly accurate one of the period. Hard to believe that a bottle of shampoo has changed all of that, but that is indeed the case. Once we began learning the value of quality products and the benefit they had on the hairshaft, those days were doomed. Why? Simple. Healthy, strong hair cannot achieve the styles of yesteryear. Many, if not most, of those styles depended upon the hair being in a weak and damaged condition.

How can we talk to the client about the damage a poor shampoo does to the cuticle and then pick up a back-combing brush and physically attack that same hair? How can we sell the client a conditioner that lays down the cuticle into its proper position and then lift it back off by mechanical means?

I remember having a salon in a building with another salon that was there first. We were both on the same water line, with our hot water coming from the same hot water heater. I approached the landlord about installing a water softener as the water was extremely hard and damaging to the hair. The other salon had a fit at our proposal and refused to give their permission. They had a legitimate reason for their opposition. They knew softened water would affect the styles of their clients. They wouldn't *hold*. Our position was that we wanted the hair to be as healthy as possible. Our styles were dependent upon the hair being healthy, and the clients were instructed in how to style their hair and also instructed to shampoo every day. The other salon performed styles that were meant to last a week, thereby putting us at odds.

In their minds, they weren't *damaging* their clients' hair, although that's exactly what they were doing. They just knew softened hair would affect the results they were after. They just hadn't learned that those styles were passé, and on the way out, and sadly, didn't learn in time, and the salon eventually went out of business, as clients drifted away one by one to more progressive salons.

There was even a saying in those days, that "you shouldn't sell your hands," meaning that you shouldn't educate the client as to caring for her hair or achieving her own style, for if you did she would no longer need you. That attitude destroyed many hairdressers and salons. And, that attitude went hand-in-hand with the feeling that we weren't *common salespersons*. Not many stylists retain those attitudes today.

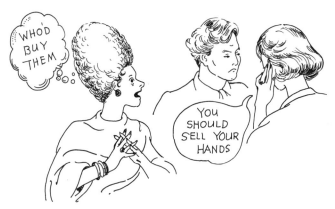

Fig. 10.2 The good old days.

It's not as though that kind of stylist was a bad person who wanted to destroy hair. They weren't, and I don't know of any stylist who sets out to do a bad job on anyone's hair purposefully. We are all products or perhaps *victims* of our experience, and we all attempt to do the best we can with our abilities. I cannot conceive of any stylist doing anything but her very best work on everyone that sits her chair. We aren't a bad bunch of people; indeed, we enter the profession of hairstyling because we want to make people look better. But, sometimes we err simply because we have ended our education and assumed we knew all there was to know. We perhaps have forgotten the axiom, "When you're green, you're growing; when you're ripe, you're rotten!"

Knowing a bit of the history of our business is important, because, as in the proper study of any history, you discover where you are and how you got there, and further understand that history is a record of change and that change is inevitable. Accepting the *status quo* is a fatal mistake. Once we begin to believe that things will always remain as they are, we are heading for tragedy. Situations will *always* change.

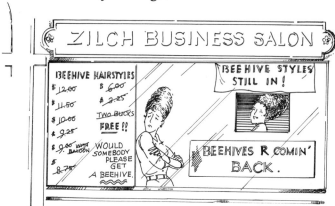

Fig. 10.3 Accepting the *status quo* is the first fatal mistake in business.

We, as a professional group, had a very abrupt change in the early 1960s, when we began to realize the importance of healthy hair. It changed the way we performed our jobs and it brought retailing quality products into the salon, never to leave it. To paraphrase Thomas Wolfe, "You can't go back again," uncomfortable as that may make some feel. You cannot survive today unless you are retailing, and the ones that resist retailing are the ones that won't be with us in future years.

Understanding that today's hair fashions are totally dependent upon the wearer's having healthy hair is an important premise to accept. It is also important to understand the place retailing occupies in our income-generating abilities. The backbone of our profession has traditionally been hair care, more specifically, the physical treatments we perform upon it. Namely, cutting and styling and perming and coloring hair. There is a limitation on this, however; a physical limitation in that we can only do so much with our hands. We are only earning income as long as we are working with our hands. Retailing opens up other, more lucrative avenues of income. We don't have to be working on an individual in our chair to be earning money. We can be selling a bottle of reconditioner, a diffuser, or a liter of shampoo, *at the same time we are cutting a head of hair.* More, we can have already sold that product weeks before, and that client is up at the front buying the second bottle while we are working on someone else. That client can even be coming into the salon on our day off and purchasing a tube of lipstick and a can of hairspray while we are home relaxing, *and making money.*

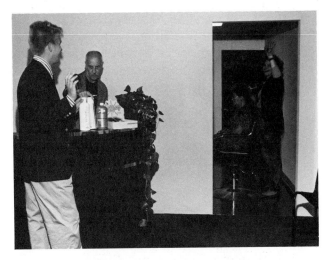

Fig. 10.4   Retailing earns income when you are
performing other services.

Retailing products opens up huge new vistas of increased income: income produced with relatively little work and little work compared to the effort expended to cut and style a head of hair. And, once the initial sale is made, reselling is infinitely easier to that client, provided you have sold her a quality product. Once you have convinced the client the product you recommend will make a difference in the quality of her hair and skin and appearance, all it will ever take from that moment on is a simple recommendation from you to try another product, provided you are ethical and only recommend that which will truly benefit her.

If your salon pays a commission of ten percent on the purchase price of a retail item that you have sold, it doesn't take a great mathematician to compute the benefits to you. If you average retail sales of only two hundred dollars per week (which is not a very high average if you are fully booked), for fifty weeks a year, you will have earned an extra thousand dollars for that year. If you have done your selling while performing a service on that client (which is probable), you will have spent virtually no extra time out of your work day in doing so. Yet you will have added a thousand dollars to your income simply by changing the topic of conversation, briefly, to your clients and to what their hair and skin needs, instead of about the new dress you bought or the menu at the restaurant you went to last evening.

And, if you are fully booked and retailing properly, you should be selling far more than two hundred a week. You should be doing at least double and triple that amount, no matter what your hair service charges are. The majority of salons retail their items at the distributor's suggested retail price, so service prices are immaterial. The number of people you see per day is the important figure, not how much you charge for their haircut. Stylists in lower-priced salons can easily out-retail their counterparts in pricier salons, if they are serving the same number of clients in a week.

Selling your clients products carries other benefits. Proper retailing can lead to selling additional services. That client who has dry skin will not only benefit from the moisturizer you sell her, but will also be more amenable to the facial your aesthetician offers. The client with severely damaged hair will not only see the immediate benefits of the right shampoo, conditioner, and reconditioner she leaves with, but will also listen when you suggest a perm for her healthier hair. The woman with the dishwater blonde hair that pays you for a bottle of shampoo that contains a coloring agent will be more open to your suggestion of a highlighting, and so on. Clients with healthier hair are no longer as frightened of chemical services when they realize you are not going to be damaging their hair as has perhaps happened in their past.

Assuming that we are all in agreement as to the value of retailing our professional products, what then are some of the ways to increase sales?

They are many and various and by no means all included in this text. Constantly observe and learn new and better techniques by whatever means available. Watch the pros at work. Drop by the giant retailers and see how they display their wares; talk to those of your clients who are in sales, whether they sell giant computers or home cosmetics, especially the ones that are successful. We sometimes poke fun at those retail establishments or home sales plans that offer cheaper goods than others, but look at their success and learn from them. They're doing something right. In fact, they're really doing something right if they are one of those products, stores, or lines that commonly enjoy jokes made about them, because, in spite of the negativism, they keep on rolling, keep on building new stores with furnishings and edifices that make us green with envy, and keep on recruiting new salespeople for their products. And it's usually not because they have a cheap line. It may be inexpensive, but the quality is usually there.

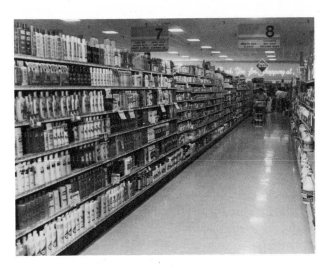

Fig. 10.5   Observe how successful retailers operate.

Walk into a major retailer's establishment and look around. Look for products that come in several sizes. Do you see what they have done, how they've stocked that particular item? Find an individual item that comes in small, medium, and large. See how they're arranged? The small is on the left, the medium is in the middle, and the large size is on the right. Do you know why? It's because studies have shown the great majority of persons are right handed, and it is easier to reach for the item on the right. And the retailer wants to sell the larger size because it increases the retail volume, earns more money, introduces more persons in that family to the product, and encourages the user to use more of the item, thereby increasing consumption and thereby generating more future sales. That retailer, or another like it, spent perhaps hundreds of thousands of dollars to discover that information. You can have it for free, simply by being observant.

Write down a favorite retail item of yours that you know to be popular with most people. Go to the store that carries it and see where it is displayed. Let's say there is a particular brand of soft drink you enjoy and you know that it is the best seller in the country. Did you have to reach down for it? Chances are that you did. The reason is that retailers have learned that if an item is popular, consumers will search for it until they find it. They have fewer problems with selling that item than with less popular items. Therefore, they place it in a less favorable spot, knowing the buyer will look for it. In the prime location,

117

which is eye level, will be the slower-moving brands, making these brands easier to see.

In fact, serious studies are done as to the average height of the demographic most likely to purchase an item. For instance, a company that manufactures or retails pantyhose will research the sex and age group of the largest group of buyers of their product and put the product whose sales they want to boost at the eye level of the height of the average person in that group. Sound picayune and nit-picking? Well, it works. That same researcher who comes up with that information will show you in black and white the increase in sales directly attributable to the placement of the product.

Changing locations of products is a theory that has pros and cons and good arguments on both sides. One camp maintains that changing the location of retail items is good for business in that it constantly introduces new choices to the shopper, thereby increasing sales of various lines or items. The other side holds that keeping a product in the same location makes it easier for the consumer to find and they won't lose a sale when he or she gets frustrated at not finding it immediately and leaving without purchasing anything. It is up to you to determine which philosophy you adhere to, but personally, I feel the former to be more valid, especially in the relatively closer confines of a hairstyling salon. In our salon, we change location of items weekly, and if someone can't find an item, they quickly ask the receptionist or salon coordinator where it is. We also notice clients walking around looking at all the items to see what new things we've added, even though they've been in the salon twenty times. They know that we are always adding to our lines and they want to see what is new that visit. After they've been in awhile and know us and our philosophy, they even ask what's new and if it's something they can use. That's one great advantage we have over a large, impersonal retail store, in that we've been able to create an atmosphere where our clients know that we will help them with information about our products, and we are eager to do so.

Selling begins almost immediately. If, during the initial consultation you notice a need for the hair, be sure and mention it. Here is where a lot of sales are made—or lost.

I have noticed stylists; even in our own salon where you think they'd know better (!), lose sales because they were *too nice*. The other day, a new client asked one of our stylists if she thought her (the client's) hair was damaged. Even across the room, it was evident it was very damaged. It was longish hair, midback length, that was noticeably lighter on the ends than at the root. Unless (and even if) the hair had been highlighted or colored, the hair was damaged. I suppose, not to hurt the client's feelings, the stylist, answered, "Why no, it's not damaged. Your hair is beautiful!'' Well, it wasn't and the stylist did the client as well as herself, a disservice by not telling her the truth. That was a golden opportunity to explain to the client that not only was her hair damaged but also why it was and what she could do to correct it.

What she should have done, was answer that, yes, it *is* damaged and the proof was in the difference of color from the root to the ends. Healthy hair won't be lighter on the ends. That could only have happened if part of the hairshaft were missing, down to the middle layer where all the hair color is.

When she returned from shampooing the client, the damage was even more obvious, evidenced by the trouble she had in combing out the snarls from the hair. She should have explained to the client that healthy hair cannot tangle, only damaged hair can, and shown her what to do to get it into better shape. At the minimum, the client should have left the salon with a good shampoo, conditioner, and a reconditioner, with instructions on how to use each and an expectation of what to expect from the use of the products.

The stylist not only lost a substantial sale, she also didn't do right by her client. What she did would be akin to a patient asking her doctor, ''My stomach has been hurting for weeks in the same spot. Is there something wrong with my health?'' and the doctor's not diagnosing the ulcer or prescribing medication or an operation to cure it, simply because he or she didn't want to be the bearer of bad news.

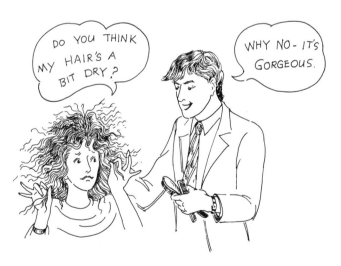

Fig. 10.6 Tell clients the truth, but be diplomatic.

You do no one any good by not being truthful, even if the truth may be something the client may not want to hear. So long as the client believes there isn't a problem, she will do nothing to correct it. It should be done in a professional manner, diplomatically, so as not to give the impression the client has done something willfully wrong or is stupid. Explain just what the problem is, why it was caused, and what it will take to reverse the situation.

Which leads to a bone of contention I personally have with certain of the manufacturers of the products we sell in the salon. While I feel we should sell the client what she needs and extoll all the benefits of the particular product, it is unethical to oversell that product and give it more qualities than it possesses. There are certain treatments for damaged hair, reconditoners and the like, that purport to repair damaged hair. Some products are, in my view, misnamed to give a false impression to the buyer. I won't name them (to avoid ending up in court), and if the product is indeed a quality product, we will continue to sell it in our salon, but we will inform the client that the name is misleading and won't actually repair the hair but that there is, in fact, a benefit to be derived.

According to my understanding of damaged hair, however, the hair became damaged, whether it was from chemical or physical means. The result is a section of hair that has had part of the hairshaft removed. Whether it is perm damage, sun- and water-damage, poor shampoo damage, color damage, pool chemical damage, or what-have-you, the result is the same—part of the hairshaft has been removed. Now, the only person I know that can put hair back on hair, once it has been removed, is not personally manufacturing reconditioners or protein treatments. To my knowledge, damaged hair cannot be restored to its previous state of health. There is, however, a definite value to reconditioners, and it is twofold. What I tell the client who could use such a product is that, "Your hair is damaged and the result is a loss of part of the hairshaft. That is why it is of a lighter color, shows red, etc., and tangles after it is shampooed. Healthy hair does none of those things, as the cuticle is laid back down against the hairshaft the way it should be, thereby giving you shine (from a smooth surface), the proper color (the hairshaft hasn't been damaged to the second layer), and tangle-free hair. (Smooth hair, with the cuticle intact and laid against the hairshaft cannot grab hair the way roughened cuticles can.) Because your hair *is* damaged, it needs the proper products such as shampoo and conditioner, and it can benefit from a protein treatment or a reconditioner or deep conditioner in two ways. First, even though the product cannot *repair* the damage, or put hair back on hair, it *can* improve it cosmetically, that is, make it *look* better, by plumping up the hairshaft and adding material to it to improve its appearance. Second, it can *strengthen* the hairshaft, so that the existing damage doesn't spread into the new growth."

The analogy I use here is to a rope on a sailboat. "Picture the rope on a sailboat that hangs loosely in the wind. As the wind whips the rope, the end begins fraying, and, even though the rest of the rope is sound, the fraying goes very quickly into it. The same thing happens to your hair. Even though your hair grows out healthy initially, if the hair has been damaged, that damage goes very quickly into the new growth almost as soon as it appears from the follicle. Therefore, there is a value in strengthening the damaged hair so that *doesn't happen as quickly*." Then I further explain, "It won't totally eliminate such damage to the regrowth."

The client is made aware that once hair is damaged, it can sometimes take a long while to regain its health, but the only way it will is to start taking care of it now.

I *want* the client to be aware of what is happening to her hair and what she has to do to keep that from ever happening again. If she wants good hair, she has to know how to achieve it.

The purpose of the above example is to point out that not everything manufactured, even by a reputable and honest company, should be taken on face value. Question every product there is and determine for yourself if the claims are really valid. Now, the manufacturers that are offering products such as the ones described, are not bad companies, nor is the product offered necessarily a poor one. It just sometimes does not do what the name implies. If it does do something valuable and worth the money, explain that to your client and let them decide whether it would be money well spent or not. Above all, be honest with them.

Educate, educate, educate. That is the key to selling. When the client is at the shampoo bowl, *tell* them what you are using and why and what it will do for their hair. Whenever you use *any* preparation on their hair, *tell* them what it is and why you are using it. That's all sales has to be. And tell them *everything* you have used. Many times, a client will ask her stylist, "What did you use on my hair?" They see a difference in it from what they've experienced before and want to know how to get that look again. Do you know what many stylists say to that question? "I used X hairspray or Y gel." That's it, period. They never think to mention the shampoo they used back at the shampoo bowl, the conditioner, or any of the other products the client has received during the service. And, they need every single thing used if they expect to achieve the same result. Everything used contributed to the result. It wasn't *just* the hairspray. The client needs to know that. What if she purchases the hairspray and gel and goes home and tries to use them over a poor quality, stripping shampoo, doesn't condition it to lay down the cuticle, then applies the gel or spray. Don't you imagine her results will be different? She may get the hold,

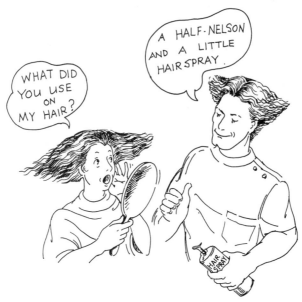

Fig. 10.7 Tell the client *everything* you used on her hair.

but will she get the shine and the condition? Of course not. She needs the shampoo and conditioner, and that's what she's asking when she says, "What did you use on my hair?"

Stylists lose fully half of their potential sales by simply not sharing with their clients every single thing they used on their hair when asked.

Clients are sometimes *begging* to buy, and we take the products away from them. Again, it goes back to not spending the clients's money for them. *Don't do it!* They are perfectly capable of saying no; don't do it for them.

Sticking with the example, isn't there a reason you used a certain shampoo and conditioner when you shampooed the client's hair? Weren't you convinced it would make a difference? Isn't that why you have it on the backbar in the first place? Why not let the client in on what you know. Clients are convinced we have *secrets* that allow us to achieve styling results they are unable to. They're right. We *do* have secrets. The products we are using on them. We don't mean for them to be secrets; we just forget to add, *shampoo and conditioner* when they ask us what we used on their hair. We only remember to mention the obvious, forgetting the other chemicals we have used.

Put the bottle in the client's hand. This is old knowledge, an old selling technique that every manufacturer has stressed for years in their selling tips. But we still forget or just plain don't do it. Put it in their hands. Once you have held something, it becomes yours. It really does.

Display your products. Put them at your styling station. Replace the pictures of the kiddies with a bottle of your shampoo. It's infinitely more sellable.

Provide plenty of each retail item in your retail area. People don't like to take the last one of anything, and if there are only two or three of a particular item left, they will hesitate to take it. Go figure. But it's true. If, however, there are twelve bottles sitting there, they'll grab it.

Ask your distributor for any selling aid they have, brochures, pamphlets, etc., and then use them. Give them away and get more when they run out.

Samples; product samples; here again, is an area that has adversaries on both sides. Some believe giving out samples creates sales by getting clients to try a product. Once they have tried it, the theory is, they won't be able to live without it, and will be back in to purchase a regular sized bottle.

We don't allow them in our salon. That doesn't mean that you shouldn't. That is something you have to decide for yourself.

My observation is that give away samples create lazy salespersons. Stylists may start out with good intentions, but it sometimes becomes easy to rely on the sample to do the selling. Instead of extolling the virtues of the shampoo and why the client should get it, the stylist mumbles a few things about it and hands it to the client to, "take it home and try it. You'll like it." And that's the end of it. Some stylists quit selling altogether, once samples are available. Some clients, who patronize such stylists, end up getting samples every time they're in, and wind up getting all their hair care items free.

Another school of thought, compromising, recommends to "only offer a sample if it is clear the client isn't going to buy." The only thing wrong with that, is that many times the stylist begins to quit selling before he or she should, and just gives out the sample because it's easier. And it gets easier and easier, until they're making a half-hearted pitch (for the record) and then whipping out the free sample.

I lied earlier; we do carry samples. However, they're not free. They're *trial sizes* that are less expensive then the eight-ounce size. We charge for them, and we charge enough to make our normal profit margin. And we monitor them carefully. If we notice a stylist selling a great deal of one- or two-ounce trial sized bottles, we have a meeting with the stylist, especially if his or her regular sales seem to have slackened, which, for some reason, almost always seems to correlate with their increase in trial-sized sales.

Assume the client will purchase what you have recommended. After you've told the benefits, ask for the sale. "May I put aside a bottle of shampoo X for you? The large bottle is a better deal. Would you like that one?" Try to ask for the sale with a question that elicits a yes answer easier than a no answer, similar to the manner presented. Some highly successful salespeople even recommend slightly nodding your head up and down while asking the question. It's sort of a subliminal suggestion, but one that sophisticated studies have revealed to be effective. Look the client in her eyes when you ask and when you tell her the benefits. Be proud of the product you are selling and act like you're proud of it. Let her see that you think this is the very best thing she can do for herself. Don't mumble and lower your head in any part of your presentation, as if you're ashamed of what it is you're offering. They'll pick up on your messsage immediately.

When you get to the front desk, ask again for the sale. This might be the time when all the nos get turned into a *yes*. Often, it is.

Recommend *everything* she should have. If there are four items you used and four items you think she should have, don't start spending her money for her again, recommend all four. She can eliminate from the list what she feels she can't afford. Chances are very good that she'll get all four, and if not, will stop in as soon as she feels she can for the ones she didn't get. That is, she will if

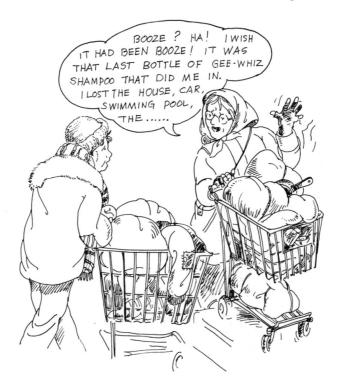

Fig. 10.8 If only she hadn't listened to her stylist and bought shampoo. An old story, but a sad one, nonetheless.

you have convinced her that all four are necessary. Let *her* be the one to say "no," however. Don't take that right away from her. Remember, you are *not* her financial adviser. You are her stylist, and your duty is to recommend whatever it is that will give her the best possible look and health of her hair. *She* knows what she can or cannot afford, and I cannot ever remember reading of any bankruptcy account in which the bankrupt claimed the purchase of a bottle of shampoo is what put her over the edge and into abject poverty.

Know what is in the products you are selling. Know that deionized water is better for the hair than the plain polluted tap water inferior products contain and that it is a costly process to deionize it. Know what preservatives are in certain products and why some are detrimental to hair. Know what each chemical in each product is and what its assets and liabilities are.

At one time, we perhaps went overboard in explaining the scientific aspects of our products. We tuned people out by explaining too much of the chemistry. There came a backlash and a situation where now the feeling is only to explain the benefit to the person and not any of the science. Perhaps a more moderate approach is to explain enough of the scientific aspect to convince the client we are knowledgeable, and concentrate then on the benefit they will receive. Instead of saying, "This conditioner will make your hair shiny," it may be better to say, "This conditioner will lay down the cuticle layer of the hairshaft, creating a smooth surface and providing shine, whereas other products may contain waxes and oils that only coat the hair but leave the cuticle raised. This gives you shine in a healthy way." There you have contained science and the benefit without being boring and have made your product different from others.

Whether you pass on your chemical knowledge to the client or not, it is valuable to at least know it yourself. How can you apple chemicals to clients' hair without knowing what they are doing and consider yourself a professional? A professional understands what she is doing and is not merely performing a service simply because that's what they taught her and everyone does it this way.

Even if you don't use your scientific knowledge in your sales approach, the knowledge you will possess will show through in your presentation, if by no other way, by increasing your confidence in what you are claiming.

Traditionally, salons carried one or two main lines and maybe a few items from a few others. There is a new philosophy coming in retailing that may go down hard with traditionalists, but you'll be seeing more and more of it, and that is to carry multiple lines, sometimes several dozen.

At our own salon, Bold Strokes Hair Designers, we carry twenty-five major lines as well as our own personalized line. Right now, we are the only salon in town doing so, but I expect there to be more who will follow our lead eventually.

There is a sound reasoning behind our decision. First, we know of no one line that carries everything needed for every single client's hair and skin. We have to carry more than one line for just that reason alone. Second, I, as well as most of you, have logged time in salons where a person came in off the street and asked if we carried a product by a line we didn't carry. We had to tell them *no,* and being professionals, we informed them of a salon we knew that did carry the product they were after. We lost a sale to another salon by doing so, but most of the owners I worked for never thought of getting that line in, even if we were getting a lot of visitors asking for it.

Can you imagine a large, successful retailer operating with that philsophy? Don't you think they'd make an effort to obtain an obviously popular line? Of course they would. That's just another reason they keep building multimillion dollar buildings and opening more and more outlets. They have discovered an open secret. You are successful when you offer the public products they want.

Sears doesn't put on one or two kinds of shotguns and tell consumers to "go fish" when they desire a make they don't have. If enough consumers want a brand of shotgun they don't carry, they inititate meetings with that manufacturer and make darned sure that that gun is in their store. K-Mart doesn't say, "Well, we've got these two kinds of socks, because we know them to be quality socks and there's no need for any more." No, they carry eleven kinds if that's what consumers want.

We've got to have what the consumer wants if we expect to sell it. Personally, I hope all salons hold off on expanding their numbers of product lines and inventory, because once more do so, we'll be forced to give up a share of the market. At least I hope they delay doing so in our area!

This is a mobile society, and people are constantly moving to other parts of the country. In each part of the country, different major manufacturers are stronger than others. We want to be able to supply the wants and needs of any client who moves into our area, whether they come from Key West, Florida, or Seattle, Washington.

Establishing a reputation as *the retail center* of your town, works in many positive ways. It greatly increases your service business, as a good number of people visit you just to purchase a bottle of shampoo unavailable elsewhere. You have already at least half-sold yourself to that client, as you've demonstrated you are astute enough to carry a line they know to be the best.

Distributors will rail against this strategy for a lot of reasons. For one, it forces them to be more competitive. For a country that prides itself on being competitive, many of us truly aren't. For one thing, it involves more work.

Distributors now have to get out and truly *sell* their lines, and help the salon owner in turn sell. When an area only has a few major product lines being sold, the distributor has it easy. They can keep a smaller inventory and spend less time and money in training their representatives. Too, the risk factor is lower. Carrying two different major lines is a much less chancy operation than in carrying ten.

I had a boss one time to whom I would occasionally suggest different product lines that offered products that were superior or did different things than did the two we carried. His argument against doing so, was that "we don't want to look like a drugstore." Well, that's all well and good, but personally, I liked the car my druggist drove a lot better than what I was able to afford at the time.

Another of his favorite arguments was that we got *service* from our present distributor, that we would be unable to receive from other lines or distributors, especially as some of the ones I suggested weren't located nearby.

I asked him what his *service* consisted of, and he said, "Well, if I need a bottle of something, Mr. X, would get it out to me that very day." First of all, he needed to update his inventory and ordering techniques so that he didn't come to a point where he needed one bottle of something immediately (a frequent occurrence). And second, the dealers we would have needed to deal with would have gotten him anything he needed within forty-eight hours through normal channels.

Another example of the *service* he was enthralled with was that his local dealer had educational shows that he sponsored. "Well," I asked, "if we didn't deal with them at all could we still attend these educational events?" "Well, yes," he said, "but Mr. X is my friend, and I don't want to take money away from him by getting our supplies elsewhere."

And that was really the crux of the problem: his friendship with the dealer, who came in every week and sat down and had a cup of coffee with him and whose kids he knew and so on and so on. All that's very well and good, but friendship has a limited place in business.

I'm sorry, but these are the facts of life. Running a business has but one central purpose and that is to return a profit. It doesn't mean providing jobs for people and making sure they have a good time at work. If you can earn a profit and do all that too, that's wonderful, but the bottom line is what really counts. All the friendship in the world, all the wonderful jobs you've created, all the good times at work, are all for naught, *if the business doesn't operate at a profit.*

Part of the reason so many salons go under and out of business is an unrealistic attitude by stylists and owners alike toward their friendships. Not only

127

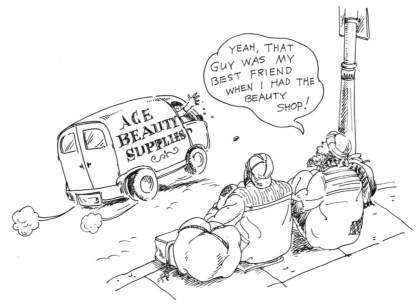

Fig. 10.9

friendships with dealers, but the relationships with clients. There is nothing inherently wrong with being friends with either group, so long as it doesn't interfere with the sound business principles needed to operate your enterprise effectively.

If carrying more lines than your dealer has available interferes with your friendship but earns the business more income, then the friendship should be sacrificed if need be. If the friendship was a true one all along, nothing will happen. If the dealer maintained his friendship mostly to gain a large share of your business, that will quickly become apparent also. It wasn't a true friendship to begin with. He was expecting you to sacrifice your income to increase his, which is not a good quality in a relationship. You cannot do business with others on the basis of feeling sorry for them. The dealer should be a businessman and understand that. If he wants to begin carrying a line you need and he doesn't presently have it, then I'm sure you would be glad to throw that business his way again, and if he doesn't, or can't, then the dealer who can will quickly become just as fast a friend as the former dealer.

Clients become friends sometimes, and can also act as a detrimental force. Most of us are in the hair business because we are *people* people and gravitate naturally and easily into relationships with our clients. This is good *and* bad; good when the relationships are positive and clients understand that for all the good times we share, this is, after all, our jobs and our businesses and there are limitations because of that. It's bad when we feel we cannot raise prices when it is clearly time to do so, because these are our *friends*. More than one stylist and more than one salon has gone under and closed their doors when they failed to even keep pace with inflationary spirals in the economy by not raising service fees, simply because they thought they'd anger their *friends,* or that they'd hear something negative about doing so. If you want to hear some *negative comment* stories, talk to your local gasoline station owner that's been in business for more than twenty or thirty years. When he started, gasoline was probably selling for about thirty-five cents a gallon. Can you imagine for a moment his doors still being open if he charged the same today? Along the way, he undoubtedly lost some *friends* when prices were raised, but he stayed in business. It's doubtful any of those *friends* would come by to donate to his cause had he kept the same prices and went bankrupt. The advantage the gasoline station owner has over us is that *all* station owners experienced the same raise in their prices and had to adjust, whereas many of us in our business refuse to anger our friends by raising prices, and, therefore, many salons exist who are charging fees that provide an income for their stylists that is somewhere south of the poverty line, but which we must compete with anyway.

In addition to the twenty-five major lines displayed on our shelves, we carry our own line of products. This is one of the best forms of advertising money can buy, and is also an image enhancer for the salon. Our products are named after the salon, *Bold Strokes Hair Design,* and our address and phone number are printed on the bottle, which contains a high quality product.

For salon advertising, it can't be beat. What happens when you visit a friend? At some point in the visit, don't you use your host's bathroom? And, when you're in there, don't you do a little snooping? Don't you notice what shampoos are on the bathtub, what hairsprays are in the medicine chest? Of course you do, and so do most other people, even those who aren't in the hair business. Even if they don't, they can hardly avoid noticing a bottle of shampoo a foot and a half away from them while sitting on the porcelain chair!

We have garnered hundreds of new clients simply because they spotted a bottle of our shampoo in a friend's bathroom and asked them about it. They were impressed with a salon that had their very own line, something most had never heard of before. In a business where image is very important, having your own product line can be a valuable asset.

Again, this is not something everyone should do, only if you are comfortable with the idea. Also, there are good companies that produce personalized shampoos and conditioners and other styling aids, and there are those that border on the criminal. Be certain of the quality if you decide to pursue manufacturing your own line. The worse thing you can do is to offer for sale a product bearing your name that is of inferior quality.

The question of carrying multiple product lines has already been answered for you. Shrewd businessmen and businesswomen have already begun the trend, one that is certain to expand and continue. Smart operators, seeing that the salon retail market is gaining a larger and larger share of the cosmetic market, are opening kiosks and retail centers in large shopping malls, where they stock dozens of lines of professional products and hire someone with a cosmetology license to manage the store. While there may be a chair and a *styling area,* in the store, its whole purpose is to move retail items. They employ the licensed person solely to be able to obtain the products from dealers and to provide the sense that it is a professional enterprise. They have seen the potential in professional product retailing and are capitalizing on it. While the trend is in its infancy now, the future is clear; more and more of these *centers* will be opening. In ten years, not only will the average salon have to vie with drugstores and discount houses for their share of the cosmetic market, but with such professional retail centers as described. Salons should begin now to counter the opposition if they want to see any of the income that will be available.

Whether you carry one line or twenty, or even your own line, merchandising is one of the chief keys to success. There are hundreds of ways to merchandise effectively. In our salon, we have a TV with a VCR that is constantly playing product information tapes. In our front window, we have placed a wide-screen TV that also plays product tapes and fashion tapes to catch the eye of passersby. Suppliers and dealers are only too happy to furnish all the tapes we can use.

Brochures and pamphlets and other printed material are next to the products and also in our magazine racks, plus we have designed our own brochures that explain to the client why we have so many lines and what each of them can do. Several of our lines are displayed with a *computer* that the client can pose questions to, that will prescribe what the client should use, after a series of questions he or she answers.

As we are in a shopping mall that promotes its businesses vigorously, and has several *sidewalk days* and other types of promotions on a regular basis, some of our suppliers will furnish outside displays and even man them during such events, testing hair and selling products for us. We don't even have to furnish personnel or equipment for such events; the dealer does it all, very professionally, and the best part is, we retain all the profits! The last such sidewalk day promo resulted in the sale of over two thousand dollars worth of product sales, and we gained several dozen new clients and the dealer did all the work!

In our advertising, a principal theme that is stressed over and over is that we are *the* retail center of our city. This consistently brings in new clients who come in initially to find a bottle of that shampoo they used in New York and couldn't find here. Once inside our doors, half our sales effort has already been done. Our personnel are trained to be friendly, courteous, and helpful; and we have a handout we give visitors that explains our hair services. This goes in every retail bag that leaves the salon. In such a client's mind, the fact that you carry a brand of shampoo she was using that couldn't be found elsewhere, implies that you are probably of the same caliber of salon as the one she had to move away from. A high percentage of these shoppers become service clients.

We also furnish local health and racquet clubs with their shampoos for their locker room areas. And, of course, the line we furnish is our personalized line!

When we do talks and demonstrations before service groups and clubs, we take along not only our brochures to hand out, but also samples of our own shampoo line. This is one of the few times we give away samples rather than sell them. We do the same when we are asked to style models' hair at fashion shows. If you choose not to have your own salon line, you can have imprinted a label to place on samples of the lines you do carry, and thereby achieve much the same results. We affix such a label to each product in all of our other lines, for the same reason. It simply has the words, "Available at," and the name of our salon, address, and phone number.

When we host our weekly blow-drying classes (more about those in Chapter 11), we always give the selected model a reconditioning treatment before we blow-dry her hair, and make sure all the attendees observe first-hand the condition of her hair before and after the treatment.

There are literally hundreds of ways to promote and move your retail items, and if you use some of the creativity you display in your hairstyling, you will be able to come up with many more ways to sell your merchandise.

Track each item you offer for sale, and if there are those products that sit untouched for very long, determine what you can do to get them sold, and if all reasonable efforts fail, replace them with products that *will* sell. Assassinate them; get rid of them. When products sit too long on the shelves, you are losing money. A factor you should always consider when estimating the profitability of your retail items, is what the same amount of money used to purchase them would have brought in a traditional, conservative investment, such as in a passbook savings account. What would it have brought if you had placed the sum there instead of in a case of brand X shampoo. If you would have made more money in such an investment, then the product is costing you money, especially when the other factors of labor costs in stocking and cleaning, shipping costs, rental cost of the area used, and all the other factors are weighed in. Experts in salon retailing estimate that if you buy a bottle of shampoo for one dollar and sell it for two dollars and give your stylists a ten percent commission, then you will realize a profit of about twenty-two percent when all the other costs are factored in, including electricity, other utilities, advertising, and so on. The profit is not as high as you might assume when you first look at it. So, if you have an item that sits month after month on the shelf, then you are actually losing money on it, and it is time to replace it with something else that has a better chance of being sold.

Thankfully, most legitimate dealers will take back slow-moving inventory and replace it with something else.

Many times another problem arises among stylists when new lines are introduced into the salon. Some stylists will cry, "But, I just got my clients to use shampoo Z! I've convinced them that this was the best product. How can I tell them that shampoo XL-improved is better now?"

Very easily. Just explain to the client that "when I recommended shampoo Z to you, it *was* the best product available for your hair condition. Now, we've discovered a better product, shampoo XL-improved, and this is why it's better." Then do so. To avoid this problem in the future, always explain to the client, that "What I am recommending to you *now* is the best available product. I won't always recommend this to you, however, as our industry is constantly working to improve products and design new and better ones. As soon as something comes out that works even better, I will let you know." Once you start selling with this attitude, you will never again feel lost when a line is discontinued, or you decide to sell something else. Your clients will understand that you are always going to have the state-of-the-art products, and that your loyalty to a particular line or item is only there so long as that line or item is the very best.

In our salon, we do the same with all of our products, even the products we use in our service work. When a perm is given, we explain to the client what perm we are giving and why we feel this perm to be the very best available. Then we add this disclaimer, "But, in all probablity, we won't be using this perm a year from now because a new and better perm is sure to come out, and when it does, we'll switch to it."

We explain to clients that the manufacturers of our products strive to always offer the best products research can come up with, but that they are also businessmen. What that means, is that whenever they come out with a product, there will always be a group of users that are *trapped* with that product—these people will forever use that product because they are so enamored of it that they will eternally be blinded to the virtues of anything else. And, so long as there is a buying segment, the manufacturer will continue to make and sell it. That particular product remains the same, but now there is a better one, and our loyalty, in our salon, only extends to any perm or product so long as it is the *best* perm. Look around on your next visit to your dealer's showroom and count the products that are ten, twenty, even thirty to fifty years old, that they are still selling, and you *know* they're garbage products. People are buying them, and it's not because they're cheaper, necessarily. It's because they've never tried anything else. They'll be the stylists climbing into the Edsel in the parking lot.

Once your clients understand that philosophy, they will unhesitatingly purchase whatever product you recommend, with the complete faith that you are in the forefront of product awareness and knowledge, and are always carrying the best available items. And, the public is used to and has a desire to buy new products. Manufacturers know this and use the knowledge effectively. Go into any supermarket and look at furniture waxes, hair shampoos, floor polishers, or similar products, and take note of the old established lines that have been around since God was a little boy. A great many of them will have emblazoned on their labels things like, "New! Improved!" These manufacturers are very astute and know that consumers will buy a product in a trice if they believe it to be better than before. Whenever an old product comes out claiming to be new and improved, sales of that product skyrocket. Take a page from the pros and use this knowledge to boost your own sales!

Talk to the retailers that patronize you and pick their brains. You will learn that one company uses red near its cash registers because red has been found to be the best color to encourage people to open their wallets and purses and spend. There is a plethora of valuable information out there that is ours for the asking. The people who staff and manage successful retail concerns are aware of many of the principles that work and usually don't hesitate to pass on their knowledge to you, especially when they don't perceive you to be competition or a threat to their own businesses.

It pays to subscribe to various trade magazines of other professions, such as retailers magazines, restaurant magazines, service industry trades, and so on. Many of the ideas promulgated by these publications can be very valuable if utilized by our own industry. And, of course, our own trade magazines are fonts of tips and information.

Successful retailing is healthy—healthy for the client's hair and healthy for stylists' and salons' success. Today, it is integral and absolutely necessary for hair styling establishments to retail vigorously. Listen, look, and learn every way existent to improve techniques of selling, and your business will prosper.

REVIEW

1. *Why retailing is important not only to you but to your client as well:* Today's hair fashions depend on healthy hair, and the products clients use determine that health. Retailing dollars are important to the financial health of the salon as well, being less labor intensive and, therefore, potentially more profitable than the income derived from services.
2. *How proper retailing builds service revenues as well:* The moisturizer sold to the client with dry skin can lead to the facial you give her.
3. *Effective selling techniques that work:* Display merchandise properly, larger sizes on the right, less popular items at eye level. Put the bottle in the client's hand. Combine science and benefits in the sales talk. *Ask* for the sale!
4. *Alternatives to traditional retailing philosophies:* Think about carrying multiple lines and perhaps your own personalized line. Use the modern technology of VCRs and client computers. Carry what the consumer wants!

CHAPTER 11

How to Build a Full Booking in Three Months or Less

CHAPTER LEARNING OBJECTIVES

The stylist successfully mastering this chapter will know:

1. *What clients are looking for and how that knowledge can help quickly to build a full booking.*
2. *How to get your clientele to build your business for you.*
3. *Steps salons can use to generate more business.*
4. *How to start a new business and open the doors to a full book even if you don't have a present clientele.*
5. *Why and how you should always continue to build a larger clientele even when your book is full.*
6. *How to take the ceiling off your income potential.*

"We have met the enemy and the enemy is us" is a quote that the cartoon character Pogo wisely uttered a long time ago. In hairstylists' cases, that saying can be all, too true. Many times, we are our own worst enemies.

My wife Mary has a saying herself that applies to many individuals, not only those involved in the hair business but also those in other lines of endeavor, when she says, "He keeps bumping his head on his own ceiling."

We are all guilty of such behavior at one time or another, in our lives and in our jobs. We set too-low limits on ourselves and make assumptions that doom us to failure.

For instance, many times I have heard stylist say, "It takes six months to a year (or two years, or three), to build a clientele." This just patently is not the case, or at least it doesn't need to be the case. Properly done, in the right setting, a full booking can be achieved in three months or even less.

I have done so in numerous instances. Having been something of a gypsy and having a *wanderlust* and taste for new experiences, I have worked in various places from New Orleans to Costa Mesa, from South Bend, Indiana, to Lake Charles, Louisiana, and a variety of points in between. And not once have I worried about achieving a complete booking quickly. How? By simply following the same procedures that are outlined in the rest of this chapter, and using the same techniques illustrated throughout this book.

Lest you dismiss the strategy outlined and think, "Well, that's all well and good for *him;* he's got all those trophies and honors and experience, but *I* don't; therefore, this can't work for me." Let me assure you that these strategies worked long before any honors were garnered or before I had accumulated a wealth of experience. And they have worked for beginners just out of cosmetology school just as well as for those who have been designing hairstyles for fifteen years.

One of the reasons most of us entered the hairstyling profession was that we saw ourselves as being creative and had a desire to express that creativity. Many times, however, we restrict that creativity to the head of hair seated before us in our chair. If you can learn to use that innate creative ability in some other areas of your business, your appointment book will fill up with astounding speed.

First, learn to look beyond that head of hair seated before you, and focus on more than what trendy hairstyle you are about to create that will *wow* the owner of that hair. Start to analyze just what it was that caused that client to appear before you, prepared to trust you with sharp instruments or with strong chemicals.

For openers, let us assume that no one in the world *needs* a hairstyle. At least not in the same sense that we all need food, shelter, water, and warmth in cold weather. Those are all truly *needs* that we must have for survival. Perhaps they are what we could call primal or survival needs.

But, in modern society, the way it has evolved, there are other needs that may not seem as basic as a hunk of meat and a warm fire, but are nearly as necessary for survival in a complex and changing world. Today, we no longer

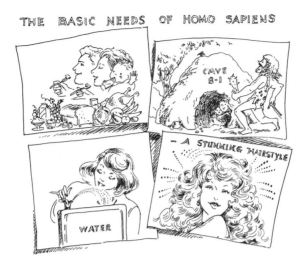

Fig. 11.1 The basic needs of *Homo sapiens*.

hunt for our food or cut down trees and erect our own lean-tos, because we've learned the value of division of labor and have invented a system that uses money as the medium of exchange to trade for not only our basic needs but also our wants and desires as well. Those who hold the largest amounts of money live the most comfortably, and this is assumed to be one of the goals of most intelligent beings.

Therefore, that great mass of humanity that lurks out *there* can be assumed to have the same needs as we do, namely, the amassing of as much money as they are capable. And what weapons do they require in that search that we as stylists can arm them with? Why, in making their appearance more suitable, that's how. There is virtually no occupation that doesn't reward its most attractive practitioners. Some occupations reward their staff or workers with higher premiums than others for a more pleasing appearance, but even the factory worker who mans the assembly line is more apt to be promoted and be in line for favorable treatment if he or she appears more attractive than those around him or her.

Naturally, appearance is more highly valued in those that work in say, sales, but personal appearance is important to nearly every job. We may view this as grossly unfair, but so is much of life sometimes, and it is doubtful this will change. Because we are in the business of image enhancement, we would be more comfortable with our occupation if we accepted the premise that beautifying others is a desirable and necessary thing to do, and did not adopt a negative philosophy toward it.

We can then see that improving appearances is a *need* most people have, to better their job status and, therefore, their income level. It is then, a basic *key* to understanding client motivation.

Sex is another powerful motivator. We are attracted to others, initially at least, because of their appearance. Later on, as we get to know the person, other factors, such as personality and intelligence, may weigh heavier than mere appearance, but most of us realize that our appearance is most important in the first contact. Sex, then, is the second *key* in understanding client motivation.

These are two of the reasons people have a need for our services, and if you pay attention to none other than these two motivators, that will be enough to build your clientele.

Sex and money. That's what people get their hair done for. It's that simple; and, that complicated.

Now, I know that 86-year-old great-grandmother who sits in your chair doesn't appear to have the same motivators, as sex and money, and perhaps she doesn't (and then, again, perhaps she does!), but there is a third reason people get their hair done, and that is pride in appearance. And that pride comes from a need deep within all of us to be accepted by our peers. That is a strong motivator, the yearn to be well thought of by others. Most of us wish to present ourselves as being physically similar to our peer group. Right or wrong, we associate the way others look, with their value systems and beliefs. That is why there is often animosity toward those who look very much different than we do. We assume they are different inside as well. Sometimes they are and sometimes they aren't. But instinctively, we view them as alien to what we are. We dress and try to look like others that we admire and like to gain their approval and acceptance.

That is the third key to understanding why it is clients enter our establishments and allow us to do strange and wondrous things to their hair. Knowing and understanding these needs clients have will help you in all phases of building your business, from your advertising philosophy to the type of style you suggest to the lady sitting before you.

Notice that I didn't include *price* as a motivator. That is because price is rarely a factor. People will pay whatever it is they *believe* you to be worth. It is your job to make them realize you are worth whatever it is that you charge. The high-priced salon is usually just as busy as the budget salon, and many times busier. Look at the salons in your own town. Let's say a basic haircut can be obtained for ten different prices, ranging from three up to one hundred dollars. Look at which salon is the busiest. I would hazard a guess that it's not the salon that charges three dollars for a five-minute trim. It may not be the salon that gets one hundred dollars either, although it is more likely. People associate price with quality, right or wrong, but that *is* a concept many hold. The busiest salon in your town is probably somewhere between the three dollar salon and the hundred dollar one, but I would guess it would be toward the higher end.

If price were truly a deeply motivating factor, wouldn't the three dollar salon be the busiest? Indeed, wouldn't it be the *only* busy salon?

And it's not, in most cases. The price of a hair service is a factor only when the potential clientele views the quality given as not being commensurate with the amount being charged. Price is only a major motivator to those for whom the three prime motivators are not paramount or for that segment of the population for which money is the overriding concern in their life. There is nothing wrong with that (nor is there anything wrong with the salon that offers a three-dollar haircut), but if you are attempting to maximize your income and potential, it would be difficult to do so if your service prices are too low. There is a legitimate place in our business for all types of salons, but for our purposes here, which is how to build a full clientele, let us give price a low priority in determining client motivation.

Considering the three primary motives clients have for visiting your establishment—money, sex, and pride in appearance—you should realize you've got a powerful ally in the media, especially TV, and to a lesser extent, the print and broadcast media. These communicators are out there helping you, every hour of the day and night. What is it that is sold every minute of the day, but sex and money (or power, which is nearly the same thing)? Look not only at the commercials and ads, which are blatantly obvious in their appeal, but also at the programs and articles themselves. Don't they paint a picture where everyone is extraordinarily handsome and beautiful and owns the choicest material goods? Of course they do! The power of those media is that the majority of the population openly covets and desires what is advertised.

Look at a typical TV automobile commercial. Do they say much about the car itself? Do you learn a great deal about the mechanical workings, how it realistically and accurately performs against the competition? A little. There are a few such nuggets of information thrown out, mostly to let you justify purchasing the car, but isn't the main thrust and emphasis of the ad usually sex? You see a handsome man or a gorgeous woman (or both), alluringly clad, talking in dulcet undertones, while romantic music plays seductively in the background, and the car being shown (in sexy red) speeds down the coastal highway, breaking every speed law in the book. The people who produce and design these ads are not dummies. They are following P. T. Barnum's advice, and selling "the sizzle, not the steak." It is difficult to pick out a slick, national

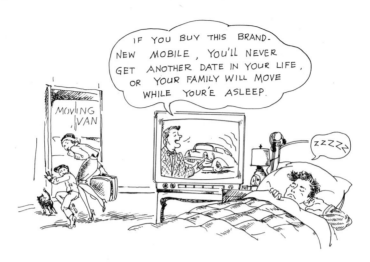

Fig. 11.2 Recognize motivators.

ad for any product that doesn't build around such a theme. That's because they know it works.

The point is to recognize why people visit a hair salon. Or buy a car. The trick is how to utilize this knowledge. Knowing the turn-ons of potential clientele helps you determine the demographics of the ideal group you will want to attract.

Here is an example of the wrong kind of advertising that will step on some people's toes. Look at the salon or stylist that is in the habit of emphasizing *price specials* in their advertising. Would you say that normally they are busy salons or stylists? Usually not. Why? Because they are appealing to only one thing: the saving of money for the consumer. That's not generally appealing to most consumers, at least not by itself. As we have said, there are those opposed to saving a buck, but if that's *all* that's being offered, the appeal is diluted. If the message is also about appearance enhancement, then the results will be better. But there needs to be something more offered than a lower price.

That's not to say you should go out and immediately raise your prices to where they're the highest in town, although in some instances that's not a bad idea. Later on in this chapter, we'll show you the way to raise the ceiling on your prices forever, and obtain an even larger clientele by doing so.

Getting back to the basic needs we've outlined, sex, money, and pride in appearance, it makes sense to understand that we need to create an image in the general public's mind that *our* salon is the place where those needs can best be met.

First, we should look the part. We should look attractive to the group we wish to attract. How can we sell fashion if we don't look the role? It becomes difficult.

I recently delivered a talk on hair fashion to a local group of salespeople from a national company that sells various cosmetics and toiletries on a home-to-home basis. Most of the ladies (and one man) present appeared very attractive and successful. One, however, stood out. Her hair was long and shapeless and if she was wearing makeup it was invisible. After the meeting, I asked the sales director about the woman. It seemed she was the lowest grosser for the area and was about to drop out. I asked if I might speak to her privately and the director gave her blessing. Taking the woman aside, I told her that I had noticed her hair and thought of a hairstyle that would look terrific on her and would she consider letting me do it on her, free of charge. At first she was reluctant, but then decided she would. The next evening, she came in after my last appointment, and we cut and styled her hair.

I received a phone call in two weeks from her manager who raved about the difference in the lady's sales and attitude. She had not only sold more of their product in the past two weeks than she had in nearly the year preceding, she was about to quit her full-time job and make her cosmetic selling job her only source of income. Literally overnight, she was transformed into a selling machine, and simply because she now looked the part.

As I travel around the country, I oftentimes observe a phenomenon in salons that is absolutely detrimental to business and it is a look many hairdressers have that I call the "hairdresser look." It is usually some semi-wild coiffure that only hairdressers and teenagers seem to prefer. Now, if you wish to build an entire business on this type of clientele, then by all means, wear it, but a more sensible (and profitable) approach might be to determine what is truly fashionable and current and sport that look instead. It makes you more accessible to a larger share of the population, especially that portion that has the largest disposable income.

The next time you attend a hair show or styling seminar, observe the looks of the majority of attendees. Couldn't you pick them out of almost any crowd and identify them as hairdressers? For the most part, those looks are unsellable, at least to the part of the populace we want coming in our doors.

The phenomenon reminds me of an experience I had while attending Indiana University in the late 1960s. This was at the height of student protests and boycotts and I was in the thick of things, marching for this cause and that, and thoroughly convinced not to "trust anyone over thirty" and all the other propaganda I was weighed down with.

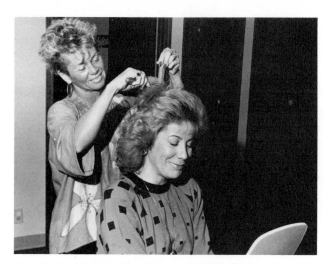

Fig. 11.3 Be appealing in your own fashion to the demographics you wish to attract.

One day, in a psychology class, a student began a discussion with the professor in which he railed against the "uniform of the establishment," namely, a suit and tie. The professor, being a pretty shrewd cookie, suggested an experiment. He had the thirty-odd members of our class go *en masse* to a popular bus stop on campus and jot down in our notebooks, what each person waiting for a bus was wearing.

When we returned, we totaled up our observations and discovered that of the thirty-four persons who came to the bus stop during the half hour we were there, twenty-seven of them wore faded jeans and a tie-dyed T-shirt. Three had suits and ties, two had shorts and a tie-dyed T-shirt, and one had Sansibelt trousers and a sport shirt. The lone person with a sport shirt was a jock, we concluded; the three with ties were administration or business professors; and all the rest were 18- to 22-year-old students. Everyone at the bus stop had on a *uniform*. What the student who began the argument with the professor (and most of the rest of us) hadn't realized, is that most of us wear a uniform of one kind or another, even when we think we're being nonconformists or asserting our individuality. In truth, we were as conforming and nonassertive as the group we were criticizing!

Hairstylists who wear the *hairstylist hairstyle* risk doing the same thing, becoming typecast as a particular type of individual. Instead of establishing their creativity, which is probably their motive, they stamp themselves as the most common of clones, and begin attracting clientele who look like themselves. There's nothing wrong with that if that's what you truly want, but if a higher income and more respect from more quarters of the population is what you desire, then think twice about the look you project.

My wife Mary, who gives me virtual *carte blanche* on her haircuts and styles, always say, "Whatever you do, don't make me look like a hairstylist." She doesn't mean anything derogatory against hairstylists; what she wants to avoid is looking like the *typical* stylist, who hasn't thought out entirely the look she is projecting. And Mary is booked weeks in advance, with all spectra of the population, even the ones that want that hairdresser look we have been talking about. Her style is always on the cutting edge of fashion, and would work equally well in the board room, a yacht in the Mediterranean, or at the lake in the summer. She looks contemporary and fashionable and, in my opinion, could take the place of any actress in any contemporary movie. She gets business because of her look, which is unfair because *she* didn't cut and style it; *I* did!

Rule number one then, is look the part, and look the part that will most appeal to the demographics you wish to attract.

The rule that precedes that is to always remember the reasons motivating people to come to a salon.

The next procedure is to get your existing clientele to work for you. We have already covered this, but it bears repeating. *Ask* your clients to send you a friend. It works every time. Don't just give them a few cards without saying anything, but actively enlicit their help. Don't ever let a new client leave without three or four cards and a request for them to send you their friends. If, during the styling, she mentions a friend of hers that could use your services, ask her for her name and address and if you can use her name. Then, drop the friend a card, tell her where you learned her name, and offer her a free styling consultation. Do this in a diplomatic way, so she won't think you or her friend is criticizing her current appearance, and the results will astonish you.

You might even take a page from the insurance business and ask the new client for the names of three friends she thinks will benefit from your services. Insurance salespeople, especially the ones earning six- and seven-figure incomes, base most of their business on this method: referrals. It works for them and will work for you.

Call the new client after two days have passed since you did her hair and ask her if she's experienced any problems. If she hasn't, and she probably won't, remind her to send you a friend. Ask her if anyone has commented favorably on her hair and ask if you can have their names and address. Send them out a card right away, asking them to come in for a free consultation.

Example A

Bold Strokes Hair Designers

Hi!

My name is Les Edgerton and I just noticed your hair. I thought of some interesting possibilities for it. Being a hairdesigner, I can see that yours is the kind of hair that sometimes poses problems for hairstyling professionals such as myself and that is why I approached you. I have an extensive background in working with hair just like yours and feel I can give you a look you will be delighted with. Please call me at Bold Strokes Hair Designers (219) 749–2366 for an appointment to discuss those possibilities in a *free* Discovery Session. We are located in Georgetown Square in Ft. Wayne.

My Qualifications

1. Winner of 16 State Styling Championships (IN, IL, MI)
2. Worked for Clairol for 2 years as a Platform Artist.
3. Guested on Cox Cable TV show in New Orleans on fashion.
4. Featured on PM Magazine.
5. Created styles for leading fashion magazines including *Bride's and Bridal Trends Magazine.*
6. Wrote hair and fashion articles for *The National Beauty School Journal, Bride's, Bridal Trends Magazine, Touts, Gambit, Dixie Magazine,* and many others.
7. Wrote a chapter in *The Standard Textbook of Cosmetology,* the text used worldwide in most beauty colleges.
8. Authored *You And Your Clients: Human Relations for Cosmetology.*

Example B

Bold Strokes Hair Designers

Hi!

My name is Kay Semer and I just noticed your hair. (The remainder of the text is the same, except for the qualifications at the end.)

My Qualifications

1. Graduated at the top of my class at XYZ Beauty College.
2. Have extensively studied in dozens of styling seminars.
3. Have been trained by the top stylists in the country.
4. Have styled the hair of models in various fashion shows.

Fig. 11.4 Example of handouts for Business Building

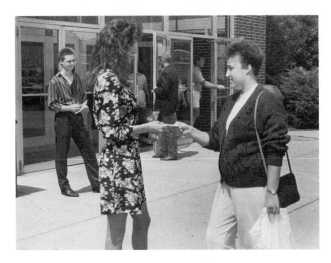

Fig. 11.5   A handout such as the example on page 144
is much more effective than a simple
business card.

Create a handout such as the one displayed on the previous page. These will help build a business quicker than almost any other method. Each of my staff has a supply of such handouts, customized for them. The one shown is the one I use. Even if you don't have a long list of achievements in the business, you can design one similar to Example B.

These are folded in half and passed out at random to passersby in shopping malls, store clerks, gas station attendants, and anyone else I see.

Such a handout can be passed out in the above manner, and each of my staff passes theirs out should they happen to be at the desk when a shopper comes in and purchases products, after they've been asked if they have a stylist in our salon. If they don't, then they get a handout. It is placed visibly in the shopping bag with their purchases, and the visitor is asked to read it at her leisure.

Such handouts are a nonthreatening way to garner new business. Handing out business cards can be traumatic to many of us, especially because it usually involves explaining to the person why we are handing them the card. Such a handout in the example takes the pressure off, almost entirely. All you have to do is pass one out and say, "Take a look at this when you have a minute, please." No more sales talk is required, or needed. Blitzing a large shopping area with these handouts is quite profitable, and easy to do for even the shyest stylist. I think sometimes those whom I hand these out to think I'm a member of a religious cult, but that's okay. As soon as they read it, they realize I'm not. The rate of return is phenomenal. I've had almost one hundred percent return in many instances.

Another source of clients is already in hand, if you have a card file system. Go through the files and weed out those clients who haven't been in in at least two or three months. Begin phoning them and reinviting them back in, or send them a card doing the same thing.

Kenneth Smith, of Kenneth's in New Orleans, for whom I worked at one time and who has one of the busiest and most progressive salons anywhere, instituted such a system and it worked phenomenally well. Each week, each stylist received a list of clients with their phone numbers and we used spare time to call them and see if we could get them to visit us again. Also, each week, we held a telemarketing class to upgrade our presentation to these clients and solve problems in doing so.

We discovered very quickly some interesting things. One common reason the client hadn't been back in was that she had had a personality conflict with her stylist. Many times she wanted to come back to the salon but not to that stylist, but didn't because she was afraid of offending the person who had been doing her hair. When this began cropping up as a reason, we began calling each other's clients and not our own who hadn't been in. This was so the client could be freer in telling us her true reason for not returning and also to make it easier to reinvite her back and assure her that the former stylist's feelings wouldn't be hurt. Sometimes there hadn't been a personality conflict, but the stylist had performed a service that she didn't like, but she was more than willing to try another stylist in the salon, once she realized no one's feathers would be ruffled.

The reasons clients had stopped coming in were varied, and in our weekly telemarketing class we brought up those reasons and brainstormed how to overcome them.

Another common excuse was that the client had moved out of the area and it was no longer convenient for her to come in. Some very good suggestions evolved out of our group and were put to use. There was a very popular supermarket nearby, which many people continued to shop at even though they had moved from the area. Also, we observed that many times, when people move, they continue banking at their old bank. With this knowledge, we would suggest to those that had moved, that if they still visited the supermarket or did their banking at the old bank, they might consider combining those visits with an appointment at our salon. Many had never thought of that and did so gladly once it was suggested.

Some departed clients were embarrassed to return, only because they had gotten their hair cut elsewhere for one reason or another and they were afraid their stylist would be offended once they learned that. Once we assured them that such would not be the case, they gladly returned to the fold.

These are but just a few of the sales obstacles encountered, but the class helped overcome those as well as several others, and the result was that we remade clients out of about forty percent of those reinvited back in. When you consider that a two or three percent return on a direct mailing is deemed successful, a telemarketing program such as Kenneth's is remarkable. Especially when the cost factor is negligible, compared to other forms of advertising.

Kenneth even instituted a separate phone line on which to place these calls, so as not to tie up the appointment phones. As his was a long-established, large salon, there was of course a long list of clients, but even in a smaller salon that has been in business a shorter period of time, there exists a viable list of potential clients who have been to the salon at least one time and haven't returned. Tap into the source!

Another rich source of potential clients are the various service and men's and women's clubs. Most towns have lists of such organization they will give out free of charge or for a nominal fee, or they can be located in the phone book. Prepare a form letter and send it to the Program Chairman of each such club. In it, introduce yourself and explain that you are available for a talk and/or demonstration for their monthly meeting. Most clubs are always searching for just such presentations and are happy to hear from you. Structure a talk or demonstration around your area of expertise. The returns from such appearances are staggering, and you need not be an accomplished speaker or artist to obtain good results.

Almost any publicity is beneficial to building a clientele, and much available publicity is free, only requiring a minimum of time and effort. For instance, have you ever seen rival hair salons' names appear in the "Business Briefs" section of your local newspaper, or mentioned in a similar service on local television? Did you think reporters went out and garnered such news bits? Not at all—the astute salon prepares its own news releases and sends them out continually.

When you return from a styling seminar, write up a brief account, stating simply that you or the staff at your salon just returned from a professional seminar in City X, at which you learned the latest technique in highlighting hair. Newspapers are always looking for filler material such as this and welcome these press releases. It doesn't mean they'll print each and every one they receive, but they will print most of them, and such notices are extremely helpful in building a clientele. Send information on in-salon promotions of staff members, new staff additions, classes attended, etc. Local business magazines are excellent sources of such publicity, as well.

Contact public television stations in your area and offer your services for local talk shows. Do the same with the local affiliates of the major networks.

The more you can get your name out before the public in such ways will increase your business and will bring you to mind when the features editor of the local newspaper decides to run their periodical articles on hairstyling. Once a profile of your salon or individual stylists appears in your local newspaper, your carpet will wear out from the increased traffic!

If you are starting a new business, use all the above methods, and also look for the other ways to attract interest. I once opened a salon in a town where I didn't know the first person, and when I opened it was to a full appointment book. How? By being as creative in business as I hoped I was in cutting and styling hair.

First of all, I ran two ads in the local newspaper. One an eighth of a page, simply announced my opening, who I was, and my qualifications. The opening date was announced as September 1. The only thing was, when September 1 rolled around, I didn't cut any hair. I sat in the salon for a full two weeks, day after day, and turned down business. When callers phoned, I told them I was sorry, but I didn't have an opening for two weeks, that I was fully booked. I even filled out two weeks of appointments in my book and scattered hair around my chair, just in case someone walked in and wanted to make an appointment. I could then point to my book and show them I was *filled up* and explain that the only reason I wasn't cutting someone's hair right then was that I had finished my last client early and was just waiting for the next one. I hadn't even had time to sweep up!

Sound devious? You're right—it was! But, it worked. When I *did* begin cutting hair, I was fully booked, because word had gotten quickly around that "He *must* be good—he's brand new and already booked!"

I'm not suggesting you be devious or underhanded, but you should understand that it's a very competitive world out there and if you don't get a bit creative, the competition will eat your lunch. In business today, especially in as highly competitive one such as ours, it's important to stand out and be noticed. It's up to you and no one else to create the image you want. Use your creative juices!

The second ad I ran was the most effective ad I've ever paid for. I had to argue with the newspaper salesman to even run it. He wanted to sell me the same old, tired ad every salon since the beginning of time had, in which I offered some sort of *special*. Vehemently, I protested and held my ground. He shook his head sadly at the money I would be *wasting* but took the check for the ad anyway.

What I wanted, was a full-page ad with only one short sentence in the middle of it. I told the saleman to use the smallest type their press had, ideally, so tiny that a person with 20/20 vision would have to hold it to her nose to be able to read it. All the sentence said was, "Your lucky number is 555–555." Surrounded by a full page of white space. (The 555–555 represents the salon's phone number.)

The phone rang off the hook. Not for just that day or week, but for several months afterward. The caller would invariably give a little embarrassed chuckle and say something like, "Uh, what's this lucky number stuff?" I had a little prepared answer that took about twenty seconds to recite, in which I said something to the effect that "I am Les Edgerton and have just opened a hairstyling salon, Hairport, Ltd., and wanted to demonstrate my creativity in an ad. If I can be that creative in a newspaper ad, just imagine how creative I am in hairstyling. I think if you'll come in and let me cut and design your hair, you will, indeed, agree that the number you just called *is* your lucky number." Almost everyone laughed, and almost everyone booked an appointment!

I'm not saying to imitate this ad, but at least be creative in your advertising efforts. Understand that the people who try to sell you ads in whatever medium are first and foremost salesmen and don't know or even care very much about your business. Most could be selling shoes or cars or almost anything. They aren't bad people because they aren't enamored of your salon (though they may pretend to be), they are just doing what salespeople are supposed to do. Sell. Just realize that what they are best at is selling you space. For the most part, don't let them design that space for you.

I was in the offices of a company that sells Yellow Pages ads years ago, visiting a friend who sold for the company. He was what they call a "premise salesman," which is the salesperson who goes out and canvasses businesses for ads. In the main office, along a back wall, I noticed row after row of books, all with the same black covers. Asking what they were, he took me back and showed me. Each book was for a particular type of business, such as plumbers, electricians, architects, and so on. Inside were hundreds of sample ads for each category.

What he did, my friend explained, was use the books as a resource and selling aid. When he hit a town and called on a plumber for instance, to sell him an ad, he would pull out an example of a plumbing ad from the source book and show it to the plumber and recommend he run it. The way he picked the ad he would show was to choose an ad that hadn't been run in that particular town for awhile. That was his only criterion, although that isn't what he told the plumber. At the next plumbers, he pulled out a different ad and proposed that one, and so on.

Don't let the salesmen design your ad! They are showing you shoes, in effect. They don't have time to sit down and be your ad agency or creative consultant. That's your job. That's a very good reason why people in our business sometimes say, "Well newspaper (or TV, or radio, or whatever) advertising doesn't work. It's a waste of money." It *is* a waste of money if you don't use it creatively, but that's not the newspaper's or radio's or television's fault—it's yours for not using the creativity you unleash in designing hair styles in designing your advertisements.

If you absolutely are convinced you have no ability in designing ads, there are several alternatives available, depending on your budget restrictions. If you can afford a good public relations or ad agency, then by all means use one. If you can't, and can't design your own ads either, then visit a local college and find a marketing student who's interested in the advertising field and see if he or she is interested in designing ads or even a campaign for you at a lower price. The department chairman of the business school will be glad to refer you to such students. Such an arrangement is beneficial to both parties. You get quality advertising copy and design at an affordable price and the student gets some practical experience and an opportunity to build a portfolio to show future employers.

If you will put all these suggestions to work, as well as what your own imaginative mind can come up with, you will be able to build a full clientele in three months or even less. Even using just one of the techniques can do it.

Let's assume that, just because of a good location, overflow from other stylists in the salon, walk-ins, or simply just because you're a darned fine stylist, you're now averaging two clients a day, five days a week. Let's also say that you've never handed out your cards in the manner previously suggested, asking the client to help you out and send you a friend, but that you begin to do so tomorrow.

When this practice is initiated, it has been observed that the rate of return (new clients generated) is from ten percent to one hundred percent or even higher. We'll assume, for purposes of illustration, that you play to a tough room, and only will get a ten percent return.

In the week preceding, you did your customary ten clients, at fifteen dollars per cut (we won't deal with chemical services in this illustration for purposes of simplicity), and at the end of the week ended up with the usual gross of one hundred and fifteen dollars for your labor. Now though, you begin to hand out your cards, asking your clients to send you a friend.

This week, you had eleven clients (an increase of ten percent) and grossed one hundred and thirty dollars. Now, following this out to its logical conclusion would have you increasing a fraction of a customer the next week and so on, and we know you can't split people into fractions, but if you will follow up on handing out cards, at the end of three months you will have increased your business ten percent per week. And that is a low average. In reality, it is almost always much higher.

The more people you gain increases not only the volume you do each week in money, but gives you an ever-expanding pool of clients to ask to send you their friends. If you increase your earnings ten percent over the previous week, it will look something like this:

Before Initiating Card Hand-Outs

(10 clients)   ($150.00)

After Initiating Card Hand-Outs

Week 1: $150.00 + 10% increase ($150.00 + $15.00) = $165.00
Week 2: $165.00 + 10% increase ($165.00 + $16.50) = $181.50
Week 3: $181.50 + 10% increase ($181.50 + $18.15) = $199.65

At the end of twelve weeks you would be grossing four hundred and twenty seven dollars and twenty-eight cents for that week, an overall increase from where you started that is nearly threefold. And, a ten percent return from handing out your business cards properly is a very low return. On the average, it is usually about a one in every three return, or over thirty percent.

The beauty of handing out cards is that the more clients you generate, the more clients you are able to hand out cards to. It becomes a win–win situation, where there is no possible way for you to lose. All it requires is a little effort. When you add the other techniques and practice them faithfully you will be amazed at the difference in your appointment book.

So now you've done everything suggested; it is several months later and you're booked two full weeks ahead, Saturdays are gone for a month and a half. You're beginning to hear a familiar lament from many of your clients. "I had to wait forever to get in to you. You've done it! You've achieved a full book! Now is the time to bask in your success and concentrate on that vacation to the Bahamas. You don't need to hand out any more cards or give people at the mall your little printed handout. You should suspend advertising. After all, your clients are starting to complain about how difficult it is to get into you, and some of them are actually very irate over the situation.

Wrong! Now is the time to really intensify handing out cards, advertising, asking your client who could benefit from your services, and all the other techniques. You haven't yet achieved success. You're like the prize fighter who is ahead on points in the seventh round and figures he has enough to coast the rest of the way. You are now at the point where success is within your grasp, where you really leap ahead of the pack. You have achieved that American business dream, to control the supply that the demand for has outstripped! You are at the point where you are going to be able to take the ceiling off your prices.

Now is the time to develop the killer instinct. Don't be like that prize fighter who thought he would win on points and ended up getting knocked out in the tenth round, two minutes from victory. Go after new clientele with every resource you have, and at this point you will assuredly have more than you had when you began. Plunge into your public relations with both feet and white-hot fervor, and when you have had your appointments booked two weeks solid for more than a month running, it is time to increase your prices.

That's right. Raise your prices two bucks. Or three. What will happen is that you will only be booked a week or a week and a half ahead. But, *you'll make more money.* And your bookings will increase again, only quicker this time. People equate quality with price, and when you're in demand and your price is higher, people will view you as even better.

The only legitimate time to increase prices, other than for inflation or by increasing your ability, is when the demand is present. When you are booked one or two weeks ahead consistently, it is time to raise prices.

And you'll lose business. People will talk about you, complain that you're "too high." Let 'em complain. Work out the math. If you increase your prices ten percent and you lose ten percent of your business as a result, you're ahead of the game. You're doing ten percent less work for the same amount of money, and now you've got that extra working time to get more clients in. If you only lost five percent of your clients because of a price raise of ten percent, you're way ahead!

Don't let the friendship aspect with your clients dictate the prices you charge. Remember when we advised that friendships have a limited role in a business? It holds especially true now. It is at this juncture that you are going to be able to remove the ceiling from your income.

Each time your appointment book is consistently filled one to two weeks in advance, raise prices. The market will ultimately tell you when you're raising them too much.

Haven't you always envied that salon owner in town who gets a hundred or two hundred dollars for his or her hairstyles? You may have even taken a dig or two at him or her, but if you honestly think about it, haven't you wished to be in his or her shoes? Well, now you can.

Do you think the high-ticket salon necessarily started off that way? Perhaps they did, but most of the stylists charging the high fees didn't come immediately out of cosmetology school and begin asking for a hundred dollars every time they cut someone's hair. They went through a process exactly as we've been describing. Each of them could probably tell you about a classmate of theirs in cosmetology school that was even a better hairstylist, even today, but doesn't earn the income they do. They just didn't know when to raise prices.

And those client *friends*? The funny thing is, that in five years, you may be servicing an entirely different clientele, but I'll bet most of them will be just as firm and fast friends as the former clients.

Start planning now to remove the ceiling from your income potential!

REVIEW

1. *What clients are looking for:* A stylist that will satisfy their needs. The most powerful motivators are the raising of their income potential, attractiveness to others sexually, and the social acceptance of others.
2. *How to get your clients to build your business for you:* By *asking* for their help. Don't just hand them a business card. Hand them a business card and say, "Do me a favor will you? Send me a friend."
3. *Steps salons can use to generate more business:* Determine the demographics you want and create an image that will attract that part of the population. Be as creative in your image-building as you are in designing hairstyles. Create in the client's mind a *need* for your services.
4. *How to start a new business and open the doors to a full booking:* Do everything in your power to appear different from your competition and create a quality image. If everyone else in town cuts hair with the client in the chair, get her up and cut part of it while she is standing. When you do an especially great style, don't charge her. Tell her that while it's "okay," it's not up to your usual standards, and that the next time it will be and you'll charge her. One successful salon I know of even had an unlisted phone number! It was amazing how quickly the number "got out" to the right people! Be different and give quality one hundred percent of the time.
5. *Why you should always continue to increase your clientele even when your book is full:* So that you will be in position to . . .
6. *Take the ceiling off your income potential.*

CHAPTER 12

How to Use Everything You've Learned

CHAPTER LEARNING OBJECTIVES

The stylist successfully mastering this chapter (and this book) will—*be successful!*

We've come a long way since both of us began this book, and hopefully, we've both learned some things that will be useful to us in our hairstyling careers. As for myself, I've relearned some things I'd forgotten and discovered some things I wasn't aware of, in talking to successful stylists around the country. While we have problems within our industry, we have a lot to be proud of as well, and our assets far outweigh our deficiencies!

We've come a long way in our profession, and, as far as we've advanced, we still have vast frontiers to conquer.

But conquer them we will. Hairstylists are a special lot. There is some quirk among almost all of us that draws us into this line of work: We are blessed with creative spirits and minds and we love people. We've been maligned and praised and we bounce back from both extremes; the praise lavished on us is sometimes more destructive than the negative remarks.

Once, at the Midwest Beauty Show, an overworked bartender told me that he "had worked every kind of convention there was, from plumbers to lawyers to astronauts, and he had never seen the likes of cosmetologists—they were heartier drinkers than any other single group!" And it's true. We work hard and we

154

party hard! We're people of extremes, which sometimes hurts us as we're involved in one of the most personal activities in life. We get to put our hands into other people's hair and change the way they look. They trust us to do that and it's an awesome trust. We do the impossible and sometimes the pay we receive is not equal to what we have done.

Getting back to that bartender, his observation has some truth to it. Think about the last seminar you attended! Being hearty drinkers is not something we should necessarily be proud of, but I think there is a reason. Mike Murray, my mentor from when I worked at Michael and Company in South Bend, Indiana, years ago, said it best. He told me, "Les, there's a reason hairstylists sometimes need a drink after work. It's because we've talked to twelve to fifteen people during the day, and during that time, we've listened to their problems, commiserated with their lives, and put ourselves in their place. By the time six o'clock rolls around, we no longer know who *we* are, and it takes two drinks to sort ourselves out again!"

There's a lot of truth to that! While I would in no way encourage excessive drinking and don't think we as hairdressers abuse that activity any more than any other group, I just wanted to point out the fact that we *are* different from others in many respects. We want to do the impossible—take an average-looking person who doesn't want to spend any money and transform her into a movie star in the space of a half hour or hour. The thing is—we do it! In big towns, in small towns, in rural areas, in all parts of this country. And we get paid for our sweat and creativity, sometimes poorly, when the client simply says, "It's okay," and sometimes handsomely, when the client says, "Wow!" And that's what it's all about, when the client says, "Wow!"

The other payoff happens at the front desk, when the check is written. That is what this book is all about. How to get more checks written in your salon by your clints and how to make the numbers larger.

Let's review what we've learned and put it all together.

First, we know that too large a percentage of people patronizing hairstylists go away unhappy. We see that it is not so much related to poor styling skills or dirty salons or rudeness, although these problems should be taken care of as well, but the chief reason clients are unhappy is that they didn't bridge the gap between the style they wanted and the style they got.

And the reason that didn't happen, usually, was that we failed to communicate well. Our TV set was tuned to channel 5 while they were watching channel 21. Our first order of business is to recognize that our professional language that we use to communicate is not very useful in that the terms are ambiguous, and we need to establish common definitions between ourselves and the person sitting in our chair.

We need to recognize that not only are we as stylists not communicating well, but also the client sometimes isn't either. What she is telling us is not always what she means. Added to our list of responsibilities is being a detective, and figuring out what it is she really wants. Does she really want to look like Barbara Streisand or is she simply desirous of negating her large nose as well, as Ms. Streisand has? We will have to find out before we can communicate with her and satisfy her wants.

What if she doesn't trust us to begin with? What if she thinks we're rookies, two days out of beauty school, raw neophytes? What if she's right? Do we have to wait ten years before we gain the expertise that will put us in control, enable us to act the part of the professional? Not at all, because in Chapter 3 we learned how to establish ourselves as the authority in the situation, even if it's our first day out of school, and we had to use two giant tubes of antiperspirant just to get to the salon. We know we have to "fake it before we make it," to use an apt phrase coined by Michael Cole, astute industry maven.

We know that the initial consultation is an essential key to establishing our authority and the foundation upon which to build our business. We know that visual aids are important, serving at times where words fail. We know that it is vitally important to a fashion industry such as ours to convince our clients that periodic change is important, just as important as keeping up with the latest dress fashions.

We know now how to avoid the pitfalls of overselling, and we know how to employ our clients as our *sales force,* getting them to send us their friends and acquaintances. We know how to get *more bang for our buck* by knowing how to sell extra services to our clientele, and how to buy the right products that will make their hair more healthy and attractive and put dollars in our coffers.

We know how to build a full *book* quickly. We know that we can't "bump our heads on our own ceiling" by listening to the negativism sometimes voiced in our profession. We know that the sky is literally the limit, once we remove those ceilings others and ourselves impose upon us.

Let's look at a new day and how it will progress with what we've learned. It's 7:45 am and we have fifteen minutes until the first client of the day, Mrs. Hardcase, a new client, arrives. We've booked fifteen extra minutes for her so that we can have a proper consultation. Everything is in readiness. Our work area is immaculate, our personal dress is current and fashionable, our hair is coiffed into a contemporary style, not a *hairdresser's hairstyle,* but a look that will be at home at any professional gathering in the land.

We use the fifteen minutes we have to call two clients. One, a new client, had been in two days before and received a cut, and we called to see if she was experiencing any difficulties in styling her hair. We knew she would be up because she was a professional working woman and had told us she went to work at nine o'clock. She was pleasantly surprised that her stylist had phoned, and, no, she had no problems; she loved her hair and so did everyone at work. Oh, and who liked it, we asked? We wrote down the names of those who had, made a note to send a card to those people, offering them a free consultation, thanked her, asked her to send us a friend, and wished her a pleasant day.

With ten minutes to go, we phoned a client who had visited the salon four months ago, but hadn't returned. Bill Smith had cut her hair. Bill was a good stylist, but the client said she hadn't returned, because she had gone on vacation and was afraid Bill would yell at her as she had gotten her hair cut in New York. Of course not, you tell her; Bill would love to see her again. She decided to make an appointment on the spot. Well, you didn't gain her as a client, but Bill would be doing the same for you when he called your clients that hadn't been in.

Then your client arrived, five minutes early. Good sign. She valued your time, and she was probably excited about coming to you. You wouldn't disappoint her!

"Good morning, Mrs. Hardcase," you say, shaking her hand and giving her a warm smile. You offer her refreshment and then ask her to follow you back to your styling area. During summer you don't need to help her off with her coat and hang it up, but if it had been December, you would.

Once back in the styling area, you pull up a chair and thank her for coming to you. You talk for a few seconds about the client who sent her in to you and how glad you are to see her. Then, you maintain eye contact with her and tell her,

"Mrs. Hardcase, I'd like to ask your indulgence for a few minutes. This is the first time I'll ever see you like this—for the first time—and I don't know any of your likes or dislikes regarding your hair. Therefore, if you'll allow me, I'd like to comb through your hair, look at you at several different angles, and ask you a few questions. Then, I'd like to make some suggestions as to your hairstyle.

"The reason I'd like to do this is that today, more than any other time, I can be totally creative. What I will have in mind is what I can do to make your hair its most attractive, whatever that takes. And, because I don't know your prejudices, I can be free to do that. Once I learn your likes and dislikes, it becomes a little harder to do so. It's the same as it would be if you were an artist and I came to you to paint me an oil painting and I said, 'I don't care what you paint, just please don't put any oak trees in the picture.' At that point, all you would be able to see in your mind would be oak trees! When I am done analyzing everything, I would like to make some suggestions for your hair and tell you the reasons I think they would be wise, and, at that point, you have three options. You can tell me you love the idea; you can say you hate it; or, you can say something in between. At least, we'll have a basis for communication. Can we do it that way?"

She's so amazed that you didn't come across in an unprofessional manner that she says to go ahead. You add, "Whatever I end up suggesting is just that— a *suggestion.* Your opinion is the one that's important here, and the one I'll respect, but I'll let you know the reasons behind whatever I suggest and you can decide for yourself."

It turns out she loves what you recommend, and even though she hasn't voiced it, you can see that it's the first time a stylist hasn't seated her in the chair and said, "Howdjawantyerhair?"

You have just entered the pantheon of gods at this point, you'll probably never lose her as a client.

As you shampoo her you explain why you are shampooing her and why you chose the particular shampoo and conditioner you did. You even have her feel her wet hair as you're leading her back to the styling area and ask her if she feels the difference, which, of course, she does.

"I can't believe how little shampoo it took!" she exclaims. "Imagine! The size of a pea! Do you have that for sale here?" You smile warmly and assure her that you do, indeed, and you will be sure to have a bottle waiting for her when she leaves.

"The beauty of professional products is that they're much more inexpensive than what you've been using," you tell her. "It's a misconception that ours are more expensive." You note her upraised eyebrows and begin to relish the erasure of them with what you're going to lay on her.

"An independent lab did a study a couple of years ago," you say. "They lumped all 'professional products' into one group, and all 'drugstore products' into another and guess what they found? They found, that as a *group,* professional products were three hundred and fifty percent more *concentrated* than drugstore items! That means, that although the cost per ounce is more for ours, used properly, you use infinitely much less and, therefore, end up paying a lot less for what you use. And . . ." (here you pause dramatically) "if you buy the large size you save even more. Each of our products has a ten percent saving each time you go up in size. Should I put aside a large bottle for you? And you need the conditioner I used if you want the same condition you're feeling now. Why don't I put a large bottle of the conditioner aside for you as well?"

The styling session goes swimmingly well, except at the end when Mrs.

Hardcase (whom you've been asked to call "Agnes" by now) expresses concern that she'll never be able to achieve the look you have at home.

"You've just gotten ahead of me a little," you tell her. "I always show each client how to do their hair. Not only do I show you, I let you do each part a little so that you understand it completely before you leave."

You alleviate *all* her styling fears at this point. "We know that all of us forget fifty percent of what we learn within twenty-four hours unless we use the information immediately, Agnes. That's normal. So, if you get up tomorrow and don't get the results we did today, get on the phone and call me. I'll walk you through the procedure on the phone and most likely you've forgotten a minor point. If we can't resolve it that way, should you encounter a problem, I'll have you come in at your earliest convenience, shampoo your hair, and have *you* blow-dry it, with my aid, until you get it. Also, we have free blow-drying classes every Wednesday in which we use the same techniques, and you're always welcome to attend."

When she prepares to leave, you hand her a prescription pad on which you've written each of the products you used and any other items she should purchase. "Keep this, Agnes, so you'll know in the future what you should be using. If you need any help in finding anything in our retail area, the receptionist (whom you have named) will be happy to help you."

Then, you hand her four of your cards and say to her, "Agnes, I'm so glad you're happy with your hair. Think about those highlights we talked about and do me a favor. Take my cards and send me your friends. I promise to do my best for them just as I have for you. Again, thank you for trusting your hair to me." You shake her hand.

At this point, the receptionist, being well-trained, asks her if she can help her find the products she needs and also suggests she book her next appointment at this time to be certain of getting in at a convenient time. She has also scanned the client card and observed your note about suggesting highlights and asks Mrs. Hardcase if she wanted to schedule highlights as well.

Back at your work area, you file the note you'd written upon which you'd noted the names of two of Agnes' friends whom she felt could use your services. You'll wait until tomorrow after they've seen Agnes to phone them and offer them a free consultation.

You clean your area and all your tools and straighten it until it is as neat and clean as it was before. You *wish* the beauty inspector would walk in now. . . .

Your second client, Marilyn, is in for her tenth visit. You've booked an extra fifteen minutes for her, even though when you did the same on her fifth visit, she decided not to follow your suggestion of a style change. It's been over a year now, and Marilyn's hair looks the same as it did the first time you did it.

Today, you're more successful because you've gone through the styling magazines and picked out a style in advance, that, while different from the way she's been getting it styled, represents only a mild change. The model in the picture also has highlights and you point this out to Marilyn. She agrees to the styling change and decides on the highlights as well. Because they are not a full highlighting effect, only a few pieces around the front, you have time to do them then, which you do. Halfway through the process, you note that you misjudged the time and will be fifteen minutes late for your next client. You notify the receptionist who will call the client so as not to inconvenience her. She calls the next one as well, as you never play catch-up with the next client. After that, you're all right, as a lunch period booked out will allow you to get back on time. You won't have as long of a lunch break, but that's okay . . . you just earned another fifty-plus dollars for the day by squeezing in the highlights.

"How long will these highlights last," asks Marilyn. "Six or seven months?"

"Not quite," you answer. "Figure about two, maybe three. At the end of that, you should still have a bit left, more than you would if you hadn't ever had any, but they won't be working for you the same."

"It won't hurt to get them again then if I like them, will it?" she asks.

You give her the proper answer. Also, you mention that a body wave would really bring her style alive. "I couldn't do it today, but anytime in the next day or two I should have some open time."

Before she leaves, she makes an appointment for the next week for a permanent. She is delighted with her highlights and mentions that her best friend will love them. You get that name and phone number and address and tell Marilyn you are going to send her a card for a free consultation and that you would appreciate it if she would recommend you to her. She was also about to purchase the same shampoo you had recommended to her when she first began coming to you, but you asked her to try another one.

"There's nothing wrong with what you've been using," you inform her. "It's still a very high-quality shampoo. This other one, though, is especially formulated for tinted and highlighted hair and will work better. We just got it in and I've used it on several clients with hair just like yours and I like the results better. It gives hair a little more shine than the other one did and it helps keep iron deposits out of the highlighted hair by closing the cuticle more tightly. You need this conditioner too. Save your old conditioner for when the highlights grow out near the end."

And so goes the day.

The very last client of the day was treated exactly the same as the first. You weren't looking at your watch, either mentally or in actuality, thinking ahead to when the work day would end, but took all the time necessary to give the proper service. You were consistent with the quality of the service rendered.

This is the highest compliment I have ever received from my wife concerning my career. She has told me more than once that, "I don't know how you do it—you've got to be bone-tired, but you worked on your last client as if you'd just had eight hours sleep and were raring to go." Heaven knows I wasn't as sprightly and energetic as I appeared, but only I knew that. The client was completely unaware of my fatigue. And that is a more highly prized compliment than any of the trophies or other honors I have yet received. It means that a fellow professional has noticed that I don't take clients for granted, the most serious crime a hairdresser is capable of. Would your fellow professionals say that about you? If not, then please change. The difference between a professional in our industry and a practitioner is that one views hairstyling as a career and the other as merely a job, something to do to fill the hours of the day and collect a paycheck at the end of the week. Let's hope that all of us strive to be professionals!

When you achieve that pinnacle of success you desire, and I truly hope that what you have read here will have a small part in your triumph, don't rest on your laurels. Always strive to be a better hairstylist than you were the day before, and the level you will eventually achieve will be far greater than any you could have ever imagined. Keep this thought at the forefront of everything you do—When you're ripe, you're rotten, and when you're green, you're growing.

Keep on growing!

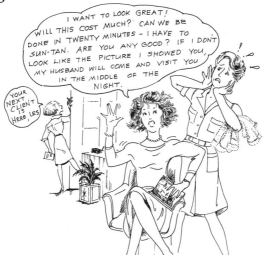

Fig. 12.1 The bucolic life of a hairdresser.